W9-BNX-591

SUPERBODIES

SUPER

BODIES

Peak Performance Secrets from the World's Best Athletes

Greg Wells, Ph.D.

Collins

Published by Collins, an imprint of
HarperCollins Publishers Ltd

First edition

HarperCollins Publishers Ltd
2 Bloor Street East, 20th Floor
Toronto, Ontario, Canada
M4W 1A8

www.harpercollins.ca

Library and Archives Canada Cataloguing in
Publication
Wells, Greg, 1971-
Superbodies : how the science behind world-
class athletes can transform your body and
health / Greg Wells.

ISBN 978-1-44340-593-5

1. Exercise. 2. Physical education and training. 3. Athletes—Training of. I. Title.
GV341.W45 2012   613.7'1   C2011-905775-1

Printed and bound in Canada
DWF 9 8 7 6 5 4 3 2 1

All photographs © Greg D. Wells, Ph.D.,
except the following, which are copyright:
AFP/Getty Images 10, 165; Martin Bureau/
Getty Images 25; De Agostini/Getty Images
116; Eward/BioGrafx/Science Source/Getty
Images 100; Bob Foy xi; The Humphrey
Group Inc. 137; impossible2possible 35, 164,
169, 188, 222; iStock 21, 28, 108, 118, 160,
168, 177; Getty Images 113, 215, 220; Heinz
Kluetmeier/Getty Images ix; Tara Norton
163; Tobias Oriwol 107; Eddie Parenti 216;
Peace Point Productions 11, 31, 33, 68, 72,
76, 77; Popperfoto/Getty Images 79; Mike
Powell/Getty Images 104; Marc Riche/
www.marcrichephotography.ca 15; Jeffrey
L. Rotman/Getty Images 6; Science Photo
Library 115; Jolyon Ralson/Getty Images
43; Science Picture Company/Getty Images
109; Lee D. Simon/Getty Images 110; Bob
Thomas/Getty Images 128; John Thys/Getty
Images 75; Steve Topham xii

CONTENTS

WORKING SMARTER, NOT HARDER

"This is my body, and I can do whatever I want to it. I can push it, study it, tweak it, listen to it. Everybody wants to know what I am on. What am I on? I am on my bike busting my ass six hours a day; what are YOU on?"

— Lance Armstrong

Almost every day I'm reminded of how old ways have given way to the new; we now know so much more than we did before. I work with Canadian Olympic-level swimmers and I'm lucky enough to be part of their support team. It may seem counterintuitive, but they spend less time in the pool than I used to when I was a competitive swimmer. Up until recently, the thinking was that the ticket to a gold medal was earned by training as hard and as much as you possibly could. Training was all about volume. But now we know there are better, more effective ways to improve health and performance. Simply putting in mindless miles isn't the best or the only way anymore. And the old way it doesn't work when you're expected to perform at a higher level more often and recover more quickly, and you can't afford to be broken down like you used to be.

By taking a more scientific approach to athletes' abilities and skills—their bodies and minds, their nutrition and training techniques—while drawing on our understanding of physiology, we can achieve more with less. A great example for all of us is five-time Olympian Dara Torres (twitter: @daratorres), from the United States. She won three silver medals at the 2008 Beijing Olympics—24 years after her first Olympics. Dara openly credits her latest accomplishments to smarter training methods, including flexibility and strength training, to complement her in-water swimming program. She achieved this level of success by swimming less than she did earlier in her career while increasing her focus on new training methods that ultimately improved her physical abilities. Dara changed the worlds' perception that age was a limiting factor in high-intensity sports like swimming. It is these new revolutionary scientific approaches to performance and health that I will explore in this book.

Athletes are some of the most dedicated, committed and motivated people on the planet; we can all learn from them. And we can learn from people who are less fortunate than us—those who experience disease. Diseases show us the flip side of the human body—the side we see when a system is broken. The science of human physiology can help us understand what is happening to the various systems in the human body when they are affected by disease. When I started working as a research scientist at the Hospital for Sick Children in Toronto, I realized that the physiology of the children with chronic disease could be understood in the same light as the hyper-adapted physiology of athletes. The physical tests are the same and the ultimate limitations to health in chronic severe disease are very similar to the ultimate limitations to performance in sport. For example, the metabolic conditions in the muscles of a person having a heart attack are very similar to the conditions of a competitive runner near the end of a brutally hard race. And the oxygen levels of a child with lung disease may be similar to those of a synchronized swimmer who is holding her breath for 90 seconds while exercising at maximal intensities. By exploring the extreme limits of human health and performance—from elite athletes to people with severe disease, we can all learn what the human body is capable of and what we can do to live a healthier, happier and better life.

Just a few days into the 2008 Summer Olympics in Beijing, one athlete began to rise above all others. Michael Phelps, from the United States, raced 17 times and broke seven world records on his way to winning eight gold medals. At the end of the competition, after all the races were finished and the medals had been given out, the beautiful Water Cube aquatics stadium was still full. No one had left. People knew they had witnessed a performance that might never be matched. And the organizers knew that

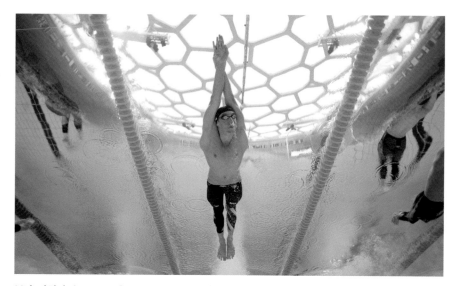

Michael Phelps' success is due to a combination of unique genetics and years of training.

this moment was special. So Michael Phelps was brought out to the podium one more time, alone, and was introduced to the crowd with the words, "Ladies and gentlemen, the greatest Olympian of all time."

Michael Phelps is obviously an incredible athlete, but the adaptations of his body may be even more amazing than his performance. His arm span is 2.03 metres wide, longer than average, giving him a greater distance per stroke. This means he has to take fewer strokes than his competitors, which increases his efficiency and saves energy during races. Height and arm length (unlike waist size) are characteristics that are largely determined by genes, but Michael's commitment to training has had a powerful long-term effect on his body that is not genetic. Most swimmers at the international level will have a lung capacity that can be as much as two times the amount of a normal person's lungs. No one has published lung-testing data from Michael Phelps yet, but I'd be willing to bet that his lung capacity is beyond limits even for swimmers. So is Michael a product of genetic talent or consistent training over an extended period of time?

Either we believe that athletes are supremely gifted (in Michael Phelps's case, with arm length and lung capacity) and therefore outstanding in their sport, or we assume that many thousands of hours of dedicated practice are required to reach these rarefied levels of achievement (like the story of Michael training 365 days in a row when he was 14 years old). It's the old nature vs. nurture debate, or in the sports context, genetics vs. training.

Exercise changes our bodies via our genetic structures, and training over time can improve not only our blood, heart, lungs and muscles but also our DNA, leading to greater health and performance. Ultimately, Michael Phelps trained very hard, and his coach designed a well-structured program to take advantage of Michael's genes and develop his physical and mental abilities to the point where he became the best athlete in history.

Achieving world-class performance in any area is not easy. It takes dedication, focus, millions of repetitions and many years of specialized training. This may seem daunting and a bit depressing. How are we ever supposed to act on the inspiration of the Olympians and other world-class performers in music, drama, business or science? All of these people trained for years to achieve what they have accomplished. What is the magic that we can extract from these brilliant performers to live an Olympic-level life? It is the aggregate of 1% gains.

THE AGGREGATE OF 1% GAINS: IT ALL ADDS UP

World-class experts in all fields train to reach elite performances by constantly improving small, specific aspects of their skill set. Everyone can revolutionize their health and performance by working to improve targeted aspects of their mind and body, even though these individual improvements are usually very small. Together they make a difference. I call this the aggregate of 1% gains. It's at the core of what elite athletes do when a fraction of a second can make a difference. But anyone at any level can apply the principle of 1% gains to get better at whatever their passion happens to be. Michael Phelps trains for five or more hours most days, but each day athletes like him will work on only small aspects of their skills and fitness to drive themselves forward, seeking that 1% improvement.

Professional Ironman athlete Tara Norton is a master of the aggregate of 1%-gains principle. She has to work on skill and fitness in three sports simultaneously: swimming, cycling and running, while at the same time eating properly, managing injuries and preparing mentally. It's almost impossible to develop everything at the same time, so working on small improvements in each area consistently is the key to world-class performance. Tara did this successfully for years. She used the 1% principle, working on physical training and specific therapy, to come back to elite-level competition despite having suffered a number of career-threatening injuries. It is examples like Tara's that can inspire all of us to pursue our passions and chase our dreams. Throughout the book I'll show you practical examples

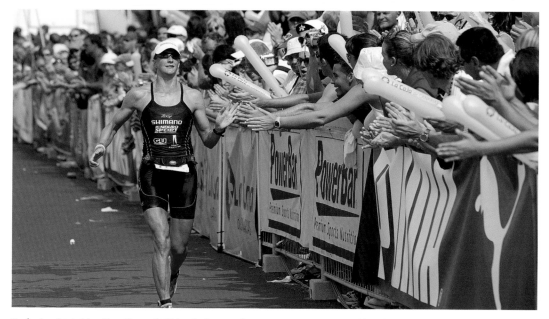

Professional triathlete Tara Norton finishing the Ironman Lanzarote race. Because triathletes have to be masters of three different sports, they work at making small improvements in various aspects of their training concurrently.

from world-class performers like Tara and also highlight the most up-to-date science to explain how the human body works, and fails, at the extremes. To help you convert these ideas into action I include "Greg's High-Performance Tips," a series of practical action steps that you can use to improve your own health and performance so you can build up your own aggregate of 1% gains!

A new study on 400,000 people has demonstrated that as little as 15 minutes of activity per day (like a brisk walk) can decrease mortality by 14%, which translates into a three-year longer life expectancy.[*]

The purpose of *Superbodies* is to help you understand the magic of the human body and to provide you with the information you need to pursue your passions with energy and health. The book will take you on a journey through the human body, using sports as examples to highlight how athletes train their bodies and minds to be able to push the limits of what humans are capable of, so that we can move our own bodies toward better health and higher levels of performance. The secrets of human performance that we learn from both athletes and people with physical challenges can be applied to all walks of life. *Superbodies* will decode the science behind Olympic performance so that you can reach your own potential and inspire those around you to do the same.

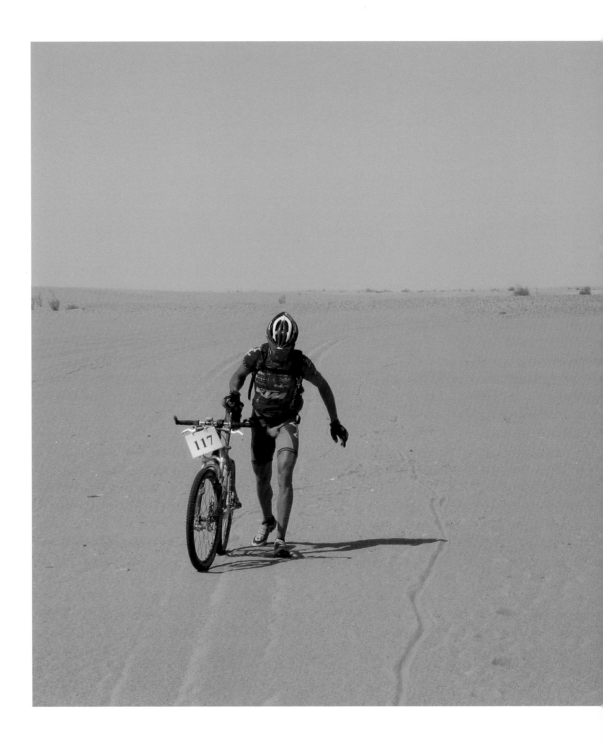

FUELLING YOUR BODY

THE CARDIOVASCULAR AND AEROBIC SYSTEMS

1

The importance of maintaining the fitness of my heart, lungs and blood came crashing home to me when I was finishing my PhD and starting my post–grad school "vacation." While completing my thesis on high-performance sports training, I sat at my desk, typing at my computer for hours each day. To fuel this intense work, I ate very well. Actually, for four months straight I ate whatever provided an immediate burst of energy. I gained quite a bit of fat tissue as a result and, by the time my thesis was completed, had put on a good 25 pounds. Nothing very high performance about that! I was not a physically happy person, but I was quite thrilled that I had completed my doctorate. Let's call this my mind-body disconnect.

I realized immediately that I was not healthy and that drastic action was required. So I got on a plane in February, when the temperature in Toronto was –20°c, and flew to Egypt to join the first-ever Tour D'Afrique (www.tourdafrique.com), an 11,000-kilometre bicycle race from Cairo to Capetown, South Africa. I was late joining the tour, so I took a short flight south to Khartoum, Sudan, and met up with the cyclists to start my journey through Africa. On the first day in Sudan, in the middle of the Sahara Desert, it was 50°c. Good thing we had to ride only 120 kilometres that day. (Important note: This practice was neither smart nor safe!)

When you are a physiologist and you exercise, your mind goes crazy thinking about all the events occurring in your body: Why are you breathing so hard? Why do your muscles burn? What training zone are you in at that heart rate? Why are you dizzy when riding? (Not a good thing.) I could feel the sweat and water being sucked from my skin by the dry air.

My heart was working overtime to pump life-giving oxygen from my lungs to my leg muscles while at the same time driving blood to the skin in an attempt to take the heat away from the working muscles and organs and let evaporation do its job.

As the bicycle journey continued and my fitness began improving—I was starting to lose some fat and able to ride well—we found ourselves cycling in the mountains of Ethiopia. Riding up the hills, we would find the local children running next to us and talking, "Where are you go?" "Pen for study?" "*Ferengie! Ferengie!* [Foreigner! Foreigner!]." Meanwhile, I was hyperventilating in the thin air, wondering how these kids could run so fast and not be out of breath. My physiologist's mind was making calculations: How dense would the hemoglobin concentration in the blood of these kids have to be to carry oxygen from the low-pressure air of the mountains in order to fuel their muscles? I was thinking that they must have blood like syrup. Simply put, the constant exposure to altitude must stimulate the youngsters' bodies to produce more red blood cells that help carry more oxygen to their muscles and organs.

Oxygen is the most important element for life. Without oxygen, we would die within minutes. Our entire cardiopulmonary system is designed to extract oxygen from the environment and deliver it to those cells that use oxygen to create energy. The oxygen, in turn, fuels metabolism in every part of the body. For example, our brain cells use oxygen to fuel the chemical processes that allow us to think; our muscle cells use oxygen to fuel the processes that make our muscles contract. To understand exercise and how the body creates energy for activity, thinking,

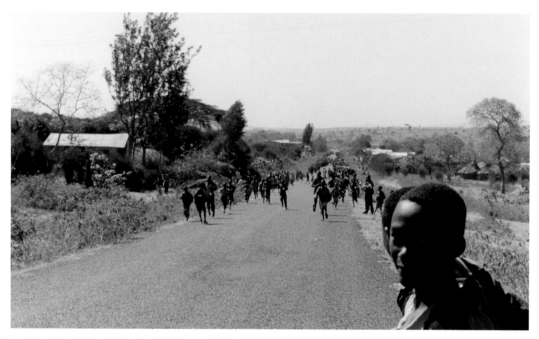

Ethiopia has a long tradition of producing world-class endurance runners. Because Ethiopians have been living at a high altitude for generations, they tend to have more hemoglobin in their blood, which allows them to carry more oxygen to their muscles and brains than the average person.

digestion and every other physiological action, we need to take a trip through the human body and follow the path of oxygen. In this chapter we will follow the oxygen transport pathway from the lungs, to the blood, to the heart and eventually to the muscles.

OXYGEN PATHWAY STEP 1: THE LUNGS

The pathway that oxygen takes to our cells starts in the lungs. The lungs take up most of the chest cavity, with their main purpose being to exchange gases from the air for gases in the bloodstream. Oxygen diffuses (passes through) into our lungs from the air, and carbon dioxide (CO_2) diffuses out of our blood and into the environment. Diffusion, or gas exchange, must happen over a surface area between the air and our blood. Tubes in the lungs, called bronchioles, take the air from the mouth and branch out over and over again. There are so many tubes that, when added together, they equal 2400 kilometres—about half the distance across the United States. At the end of the bronchioles are tiny air sacs called alveoli. This is where gas exchange takes place. The lungs have about 400 million of these sacs, with a total surface area of 70 square metres (large enough to cover a tennis court).

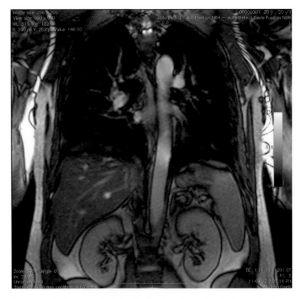

An **MRI** *of a healthy chest cavity showing the aorta, the lungs, the liver and the kidneys. Although most people think of lungs as open sacs, they are actually dense blocks of tissue filled with lots of blood.*

Our lungs, which look and feel like sponges, are attached to the inside of the rib cage on the sides and top and to the diaphragm muscle on the bottom. When we breathe, the muscles of the rib cage and the diaphragm contract to expand the space inside the chest cavity. This process creates negative pressure inside the body and sucks air into the lungs (assuming the mouth and nose are open). The opposite happens when we exhale—the muscles relax and the lungs pull the rib cage and diaphragm back in, an action that pushes air out of the lungs. Breathing is just the contraction and relaxation of muscles, a process that either pulls air out of the lungs or pushes it into them. The movement of air keeps gases and fresh air moving across the surface of all the alveoli in the lungs. This movement helps with oxygen uptake and carbon dioxide removal.

Most people breathe about 11,000 litres of air in one day, but an athlete who is exercising at a maximum level can breathe up to 200 litres in one minute—the equivalent of 288,000 litres a day. We can increase our ventilation by either increasing our breathing frequency (from 8 to 10 breaths per minute at rest to 40 to 60 breaths per minute during exercise) or increasing our tidal or normal breath volume (from 0.5 litres per breath at rest to 5 litres per breath during exercise). The body has a huge capacity to adapt to instant changes in oxygen demands.

Since the air we breathe is not always clean, the body has a built-in filter system that consists of millions of tiny "hairs," called cilia, which line the airways. It has been suggested that cilia are among the first structures to develop in the fetus and that the appropriate movement of cilia is important in the proper development and alignment of organs in the human embryo. These cilia, in partnership with mucus (yes, *that* kind of mucus) secreted by cells that line the airways, capture most particles that we inhale and sweep them back up into our throats, where we either cough them out or swallow them.

There is, however, a rare and incurable genetic disease called primary ciliary dyskinesia (PCD), which causes cilia movement to be unsynchronized and inefficient. In people with PCD, cilia are unable to sweep out particles and bacteria, so infections of the lungs and airways develop. These infections can lead to permanent lung damage, and in severe cases patients must undergo a lung transplant. Interestingly, about half the patients with PCD have reversed internal organs, as in a mirror image (this condition is technically called *situs invertus*); for example, the heart is found on the right rather than the left side of the chest. We don't know what causes this reversal to happen, only that a mutation in the genes of 0.01% of the population results in the anomaly.

PCD is now the subject of intense research, and our team at the Hospital for Sick Children in Toronto has recently published important data showing that children with PCD have thinner bones than kids with cystic fibrosis (CF), another rare lung disease. (In CF, thick mucus is hard to clear from the lungs, which become a breeding ground for bacteria—leading to long-term [chronic] lung infection, inflammation and, eventually, permanent lung damage.) The inflammation that comes with lung disease affects other organs in the body as well as muscles. Since bones and muscles seem to be affected, exercise may prove to be a terrific treatment for people with PCD, as it is for those with CF.

While lung diseases like PCD or CF can impair the person's ability to exercise, physical training and genetic predisposition (getting the right genes from your parents) can create extraordinarily positive adaptations in the human body. Lungs have most likely been pushed to their furthest limit in the sport of free diving. Free diving, also called breath-hold diving,

⚜ GREG'S HIGH-PERFORMANCE TIPS
YOU CAN TRAIN YOUR LUNG MUSCLES

In respiratory muscle training, a relatively new form of training, people either breathe at a higher than normal level (hyperpnea) for a period of time or breathe against a resistance. Research in this area has demonstrated that the respiratory muscles adapt to specific muscle training. For example, the endurance capacity of the breathing muscles can be increased through hyperpnea training, and their strength can be increased through resistance training.

Check out PowerLung (www.powerlung.com) for respiratory muscle strength training (just add the PowerLung to your normal weights routine; for example, three sets of 8–12 reps). Or see SpiroTiger (www.fact-canada.com/SpiroTiger/spirotiger-respiratory-trainer.html) if you wish to try respiratory muscle endurance training. Research on rowers has shown that you can use either technique before working out to improve your performance during exercise. Rowers were asked to perform breathing against resistance (e.g., lifting weights) while inhaling for 30 repetitions and then head out on the water to warm up. A performance test revealed a significant improvement when rowers added breathing exercises to their warm-up protocol.

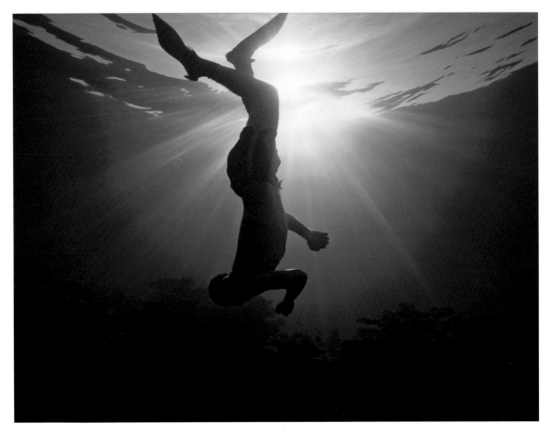

Free divers demonstrate the incredible adaptability of the human respiratory system. With training, an athlete's lung capacity can reach 8 litres—double the capacity of the average person.

has its origins in Japan and Korea, where for more than two thousand years men and women have been diving in the ocean for food and pearls. Free diving has recently taken hold as a sport, and people now practise and compete to see who can dive deepest into the ocean in a single breath and return to the surface without losing consciousness. The current world record for diving with no equipment is 95 metres, while competitors using fins have been able to dive to a record depth of 124 metres. No-limit free diving (in which competitors can use any equipment) has produced a world-record depth of 214 metres.

If you dive deep into the ocean, your body goes through extraordinary adaptations. Deep-sea divers have trained themselves to hold their breath for several minutes at a time—the record now stands at over 10 minutes for static apnea (no breathing) and a bit longer than four minutes for free

DISTANCE PER BREATH

People are always looking for ways to make their workouts more challenging and interesting. You can try changing your intensity for a period of time or adding some hills if you're running. You can also try changing your breathing pattern. For a new challenge, try slowing down or speeding up your breathing while exercising. If you are doing some short sprints, try holding your breath for a few seconds during the sprint. Being aware of your breathing and taking control of it can be difficult and make for a tough workout. Start slowly by changing your breathing pattern for a few seconds at a time. Remember to slow down or stop if you feel dizzy.

With competitive swimmers, we have used this idea to create a new training technique called "distance per breath." Instead of trying to swim with longer strokes (distance per stroke), we ask our athletes to swim with longer intervals between breaths (breathing every 2, 3, 4, 5, 7 or 9 strokes). I've found that this method helps technique and physiology. More specifically, when swimmers can focus only on their stroke and their technique is not changed by turning the head to breathe, their underwater hand and arm mechanics tend to be better. This helps "groove the stroke" and, as the swimmers get fitter, the breath control actually helps them relax while swimming. From a physiological perspective, holding your breath during exercise increases the concentration of carbon dioxide in the blood. This helps blood vessels in the muscles dilate (open up) so that blood flow to and from the exercising muscles increases. I have found that adding some breath-holding exercises to a warm-up can speed the physiological activation process.

Breathing is equally important in other sports, although the link may not be as obvious as in swimming. Research has shown that in most sports with a rhythmic component (e.g., running, swimming, cycling and paddling sports), breathing pattern is linked to the movement. This is called entrainment. It is therefore helpful to work on integrating a good breathing rhythm into the technique of the movement and to keep the breathing as relaxed and efficient as possible.

diving. These divers expose themselves to low oxygen and high carbon dioxide so many times that their chemoreceptors become desensitized. Chemoreceptors are structures in the aorta (peripheral chemoreceptors) and on the surface of the brain stem (central chemoreceptors) that "taste" chemical levels in the blood and cerebrospinal fluid.

If you hold your breath, you stop gas exchange in your lungs, causing oxygen levels to drop and carbon dioxide levels to rise. The chemoreceptors notice this change and send signals to the brain, telling you to breathe. You can experience this effect if you try to hold your breath for a minute or so. After a few seconds, you will start to feel the urge to breathe. This feeling is the result of your chemoreceptors sensing rising CO_2 levels and sending emergency "breathe harder" signals to your brain. In my PhD research, I studied the effect of training on chemoreception in competitive swimmers and showed that they too can desensitize their peripheral chemoreceptors. We think that this desensitization benefits swimmers by training away the urge to breathe. This allows them to hold longer strokes without rushing to the next breath, and to make more efficient turns because they can stay below the surface of the water longer after pushing off the wall. The incredible distances Michael Phelps swims underwater on his turns went a long way toward helping him win eight gold medals in the 2008 Beijing Olympics. This is the greatest performance by an Olympian in a single Games.

To Breathe or Not to Breathe

Traditional thinking—reflected in many exercise physiology textbooks—suggests that the lungs and the respiratory system in general do not present a limiting factor in exercise. Most texts suggest that you can't train the respiratory system either, and since the lungs are not a limiting factor, why would you want to? As with most preconceived notions about the limits of the human body, this one is proving to be untrue. We just have to look at how far free divers have pushed the limits of how big and efficient the lungs can become. A typical person can inhale 2.5 to 4 litres of air per breath. Free divers train for years to increase their lung capacity to between 7 and 8 litres. This capacity is very important because if a diver descends to 100 metres below the ocean surface, the pressure will decrease the gas volume inside the lungs to less than 0.8 litres. (This is due to Boyle's Law, which describes the relationship between the pressure and volume of a gas.) So the more air that can be taken into the lungs before the dive begins, the greater the amount of oxygen available to the diver underwater. That's because the volume of air in the lungs decreases as the pressure increases.

Free divers descend well below the depths that normal scuba divers attempt. For example, the world record for no-limit free diving is now more than 200 metres, but scuba divers will usually not exceed a depth of about 30–40 metres. Free divers also ascend as quickly as possible—something that scuba divers are taught never to do because they will get the "bends." The bends, or decompression sickness, occur when dissolved gases begin to bubble out of the blood—like opening a can of pop—as a scuba diver approaches the surface. If divers ascend slowly, then the gases pass slowly out of the blood and into the lungs, and are exhaled. But if scuba divers ascend too quickly, the gases bubble out into the blood and can result in excruciating pain and even death.

Interestingly, free divers don't get the bends. The pressure of the ocean compresses the air in their lungs as they descend, but exposure time is not very long. Because the exposure to high pressure is brief, there isn't enough time for the gases to be pushed out of the lungs and into the blood. As well, the pressure may push fluid out of the blood and into the lungs, creating a liquid barrier between the air in the lungs and the blood. This barrier slows down gas uptake by the blood. So, even though free divers exceed the limits of scuba divers and descend and ascend quickly, they don't encounter the physiological problems that scuba divers need to avoid. Repeated free dives may cause some decompression sickness, as is reported for Korean ama divers. (Ama diving is a 2000-year-old tradition in which women dive into the ocean to collect pearls while holding their breath.[1]) But repeated training at taking big breaths and holding them during exercise has allowed free divers to train their respiratory systems to do things that would have been considered impossible as little as 20 years ago.

Getting oxygen into the blood to fuel our muscles and brain when we're at rest is a complicated process. Getting oxygen in during exercise is even more challenging. Dr. Jerome Dempsey and his colleagues at the University of Wisconsin have done some interesting research on the interaction between breathing and blood flow.[2] What they have been able to show is that respiratory muscles have nerve connections to the brain, called type III and IV afferent nerves. These nerve fibres sense the physiological stress of the muscles that help us breathe and adjust blood flow within the body to make it a priority for oxygen in the blood to be delivered to the muscles that control breathing. The breathing muscles make up about 15% of the total muscle mass of our bodies, so they can demand a significant percentage of the total oxygen delivery via the blood during exercise. Dr. Dempsey calls this adjustment of blood flow by the nervous system the muscle sympathetic nervous system activation (MSNA) hypothesis.

GREG'S HIGH-PERFORMANCE TIPS

HOW DO I KNOW HOW HARD I AM EXERCISING?

Dr. Robert Goode of the University of Toronto has developed a practical test to see where you are on your exercise intensity curve. He suggests that if you're able to carry on a conversation while exercising, you are below your first threshold and are using your aerobic system. If you increase your intensity to the point where you can hear yourself breathing, you are between your first and second thresholds and are using a combination of aerobic and anaerobic metabolism. Finally, if you are exercising so intensely that you can no longer carry on a conversation, you are above your second threshold and are relying increasingly on anaerobic metabolism to fuel your exercise.

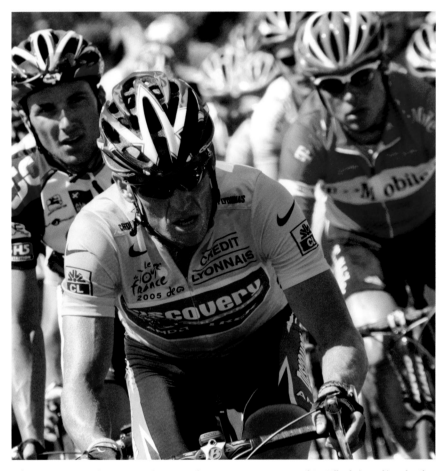

A famous moment in the 2001 Tour de France when Lance Armstrong passed Jan Ullrich (in pink) in the Alps.

The way this process works is simple. The harder our respiratory muscles work to fuel gas exchange for exercise, the greater the amount of blood that is redirected to our breathing muscles from the peripheral muscles (e.g., the arms and legs) that are doing the exercise. I think the 2001 Tour de France provided one of the best examples. Lance Armstrong and Jan Ullrich were on a very difficult climb, with Armstrong gradually and steadily increasing the pace. Ullrich was able to stay near Armstrong's back wheel for a while. Armstrong, however, was eventually able to ride away—but only after taking a look back to see how Ullrich was feeling. This moment, when Armstrong turned to check on Ullrich, is called "the look." Physiologically, what happened was this: As Armstrong increased the pace of the climb, the oxygen demand on the cyclists' muscles also increased. Their muscles started extracting more oxygen from their blood, causing the level of oxygen in the blood to drop. This drop in oxygen, along with the increased carbon dioxide (CO_2) production by the working muscles and subsequent CO_2 dump into the blood, signalled the chemoreceptors to start "diving breathing." Therefore, the cyclists' breathing increased. Breathing was increased by the work of the respiratory muscles—the intercostals (which help us exhale) between the ribs and the diaphragm, and the diaphragm and the abdominals. This is the critical moment. Because Armstrong's fitness level was slightly better than Ullrich's, his leg muscles were using just a bit less oxygen to sustain the climb. As a result, Armstrong's breathing system didn't have to work as hard, so his breathing muscles were a bit more relaxed. At this breaking point, when Armstrong attacked and sprinted to open up a gap, he was able to call on his energy reserve. Ullrich was unable to respond because his breathing muscles were stealing blood from his legs to fuel his breathing.

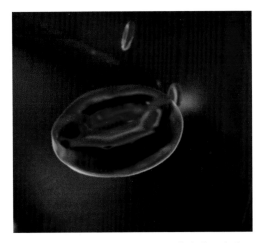

Red blood cells carry oxygen to tissues in the body and take carbon dioxide from tissues back to the lungs. Exercise and proper nutrition can increase the number of red blood cells in the body, which can help prevent fatigue.

In 2005, Dr. Ed Coyle published some controversial physiological-testing results from Lance Armstrong. The most interesting finding was that most of Lance's test results were typical of an elite cyclist: a maximum heart rate of about 200 beats per minute (b/m), and blood lactate thresholds that occurred at about 85% of his maximum aerobic power (VO_{2max}). However, the fascinating adaptation that allowed Lance to excel in the critical climbing stages was that he produced very little lactic acid (6.3 to 7.5 millimoles/litre) at high-intensity exercise levels near the end of the VO_{2max} testing. (Lactic acid is a complicated topic that I'll explore in Chapter 2.) Since lactic acid levels in the blood can cause us to breathe harder, and because Lance's blood lactate levels were so low at maximum exercise, it's possible that lower lactate levels did not drive his breathing rate as high as his competitors'; therefore, Lance was not at risk of the negative effects of the MSNA hypothesis (where blood would be stolen from the cycling legs to fuel the breathing muscles). Basically, Lance Armstrong could breathe in a relaxed, controlled manner while his competitors were hyperventilating.

HOW DO I INCREASE MY BLOOD IRON LEVELS?

The body requires iron to deliver oxygen to all tissues and produce energy at the cellular level. Oxygen binds to hemoglobin in the blood, and iron is a key component of the hemoglobin molecule.

Factors that can deplete iron levels include:

- heavy training, especially endurance exercise
- menstruation
- vegetarianism or veganism
- high-carbohydrate/low-protein diets
- diets high in processed and refined foods

- high consumption of bran, wheat or soy products
- consumption of coffee and tea
- use of antacids (e.g., Tums, Rolaids)
- presence of parasites or the H.pylori bacteria

Deficiency symptoms include:

- diminished exercise capacity
- general fatigue and weakness

- a desire to sleep more

Ways to Increase Iron Intake and Absorption

Consume foods high in iron such as red meats, dark green vegetables, quinoa, beans, lentils, nuts and seeds. Absorption of iron from vegetables is improved with simultaneous meat consumption. Include lots of vitamin C–containing foods since this vitamin is the most potent iron-enhancer we know. Avoid excessive consumption of tea, coffee, energy drinks (e.g., Red Bull). Use an iron supplement if prescribed by your doctor. Do not take iron supplements with calcium or vitamin E supplements. To enhance iron absorption even further, add some real lemon/lime juice or vinegar to your water.

Foods That Are High in Iron

Here is a list of foods that are high in iron. Note that heme sources of iron are more easily absorbed than non-heme sources.

Heme sources. Organ meats (liver, kidney, heart); lean red meats (steak, ground beef, veal, bison, lamb); poultry (turkey [dark meat], duck); shellfish (clams, mussels, oysters, sardines). Certified organic or wild game is recommended for meat and poultry whenever possible.

Non-heme sources. Legumes (lima, kidney and navy beans, chick peas, lentils); vegetables (parsley, spinach, radishes, mustard and turnip greens, endive, Swiss chard, shiitake mushrooms, asparagus, leeks, Brussels sprouts); quinoa; dried fruit (apricots, prunes, raisins, currants, dates, figs); avocado; muesli; nuts and seeds (almonds, Brazil nuts, cashews, pistachios, walnuts, pumpkin and sunflower seeds).

Iron is one of the most difficult minerals to absorb, although vitamin C helps to increase absorption. Foods that are high in vitamin C include oranges, tomatoes, berries, broccoli, mangos, apricots, watermelon, bell peppers, cabbage, grapefruit, spinach, lemons, limes, peaches and nectarines.

Source: Trionne Moore, BA RHN, www.trionne.ca

OXYGEN PATHWAY STEP 2: THE BLOOD

The pathway that oxygen takes continues from the lungs into the red blood cells. Red blood cells, or erythrocytes, are specialized cells that are present in the blood. (Other components of blood include white blood cells and the clear fluid called plasma.) The percentage of the blood that is made up of red blood cells, called hematocrit, is normally 35 to 45%. If an athlete's hematocrit is over 50%, then he or she is temporarily suspended from competition because of the increased risk of heart attack or aneurism. Basically the blood is too thick, and clots may form when blood cells bump into each other and start to clump together. These clots can then travel through the body and may end up blocking small blood vessels in the heart muscle, the lung capillaries or even the brain.

The primary function of the red blood cells is to transport oxygen from the lungs to the tissues and remove carbon dioxide from the body. Red blood cells are able to perform this function because they contain hemoglobin molecules made up of proteins and iron. Each hemoglobin molecule can bond to and transport four oxygen molecules. The amount of oxygen that is carried by the blood depends on the pressure of oxygen (PO_2) in the atmosphere around us. Thus, in the lungs, where the partial pressure of oxygen is high because of the fresh air that's present, hemoglobin binds easily to oxygen, and the red blood cells become saturated with it. The opposite is true within the muscles because the metabolism of the body uses up the oxygen that's present.

The total mass of red blood cells in the circulatory system is regulated within very narrow limits. New red blood cells (reticulocytes) are produced in the bone marrow. The principal factor that stimulates red blood cell formation is the circulating hormone erythropoietin (EPO). EPO is secreted in response to low oxygen levels (e.g., when you ascend in altitude) and also in response to exercise. Thus, exercise can increase the percentage of new red blood cells in the body. New red blood cells contain more hemoglobin than older ones and thus can carry greater amounts of oxygen.

The best example of how sensitive the body is to oxygen levels and how the human body can change in response to a different environment is found in high-altitude mountaineering—climbing Mount Everest, for example. At increasing distances above sea level, the barometric pressure, temperature and relative humidity decrease. The decrease in barometric pressure results in a decrease in the partial pressure of atmospheric gases. This means that when you move from sea level to higher altitude, the

HUMAN EVOLUTION AND ADAPTATION TO ALTITUDE

Ethiopia is the cradle of civilization. From there, over time, humans migrated through Asia, over land bridges to North America and down to South America. Along the way, small isolated groups moved to areas of elevation. Some of those who stayed in Ethiopia settled in the highlands, likely over 100,000 years ago. Approximately 40,000 to 25,000 years ago, others settled in the Himalayas. More recently, about 10,000 to 4000 years ago, yet others settled in the Andes mountains.

Over successive expeditions, Dr. Joe Fisher at the University of Toronto has been tracking particular aspects of each group's adaptation to altitude. Himalayans and Andeans are readily accessible for study but, for reasons of local politics and geography, Ethiopian highlanders have been infrequently researched. In one such rare expedition to Ethiopia in 2005, Dr. Fisher took measurements that indicated these highlanders were not as distressed by the lack of oxygen and breathed less in their environment than the Andean and Himalayan highlanders (or the lowlanders acclimatized to the altitude). He therefore strongly suspects that Ethiopians who have lived at a high altitude for generations have developed some sort of genetic adaptation as a result of natural selection. Whereas these adaptations have been found in animals such as mice, llamas and bar-headed geese, none has been reported in humans—yet

total pressure of the atmosphere decreases because the weight of the air at high altitudes is lower. At sea level, for example, the weight of the Earth's atmosphere exerts a barometric pressure equal to about 760 mmHg (millimeters of Mercury). This is not the case, however, at the top of Mount Everest, where the barometric pressure is only 250 mmHg. The percentage concentration of each gas that makes up air stays the same—but the weight of the atmosphere decreases. For example, the percentage of oxygen in the air is the same at sea level and at the top of Everest—it is always about 21% (the rest is mostly nitrogen). This means that although there's as much oxygen in the air, there's less pressure in the air in our lungs to drive oxygen into our blood. As a result, our blood can become de-saturated of oxygen if we go to a high altitude. If you were transported from sea level and dropped off on the top of Mount Everest, you would collapse, lose consciousness and probably die relatively quickly. People are now able to climb Everest with some regularity because the body can adapt and respond to changes in its environment.

Exposure to altitude has been shown to affect nearly every physiological system in the human body. The first adaptation that's seen when people ascend to altitude is an increase in breathing. This is sometimes called the hypoxic ventilatory response (HVR). The lower levels of oxygen in the blood increase the sensitivity of our chemoreceptors, which signal our brain to increase breathing. After some time, the increased breathing blows off some of the excess carbon dioxide in our blood, and breathing eventually returns to normal levels. The lower carbon dioxide levels also make our blood less acidic than normal. The enzymes in our body that

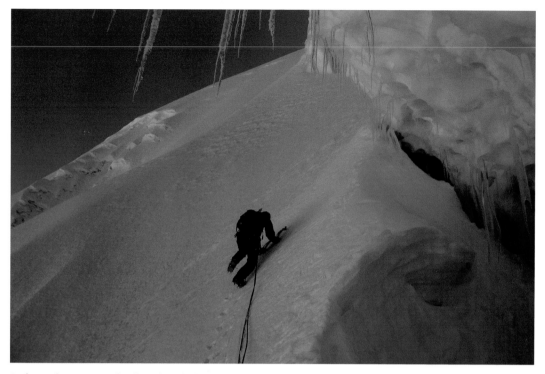

Professional mountain guide Lilla Molnar climbing in Peru. Cold decreases blood flow to the extremities, while low air pressure decreases the body's ability to absorb oxygen.

enable reactions work only within a certain acidity zone. If our bodies become too acidic, as when we do sprint exercise, or too basic, as when we hyperventilate for hours or days when exposed to altitude, then our muscles begin to encounter problems. This may be why people experience muscle cramps during the first days and weeks at altitude.

I experienced all the above when I flew from Lima, Peru, which is at sea level, to Cuzco, which is 4000 metres above sea level. I was on my way to hike the Inca Trail through the Andes to the city of Machu Picchu. Walking toward the terminal after we landed, I nearly passed out. The sudden ascent to altitude left me breathless and very dizzy. I now realize that the sensation of breathlessness was triggered by my peripheral chemo-receptors sending alarm signals that the oxygen level in my blood was low. My dizziness was caused by the fact that my breathing was much quicker, so I was blowing off all my carbon dioxide. Low carbon dioxide levels cause vasoconstriction in the brain—this means that all the small blood vessels in my brain were decreasing in diameter and that blood flow was decreasing as well. Over the next three or four days, I gradually began to feel better. By the end of the trek to Machu Picchu, I felt fantastic.

Interestingly, a high HVR seems to protect climbers from acute mountain sickness and from pulmonary (lung) and cerebral (brain) edema (bleeding) while at altitude. The thinking is that the higher-breathing response to low oxygen works to keep the body closer to normal levels, even though the environmental oxygen levels are low. Researchers are not sure if this adaptation is trained or if certain people are born with different chemosensitivities and HVRs. At the other end of the spectrum are synchronized swimmers who, despite performing repeated breath-holds underwater, where oxygen levels drop, have very low chemosensitivity. Researchers including Dr. James Duffin at the University of Toronto suggest that this is because synchro swimmers (and competitive swimmers generally) have trained away their sensitivity to carbon dioxide. And since both oxygen and carbon dioxide are sensed by the same receptor—the peripheral chemoreceptors—swimmers have a lower breathing response to changes in these gases.

Spending time at altitude has profound and well-researched effects on the blood. Immediately on ascent to altitude, oxygen levels in the blood decrease. This change is sensed by the kidneys, which filter blood and control the release of EPO. EPO remains increased for three to five days after ascent to altitude, then slowly returns to normal. It circulates throughout the body and stimulates the bone marrow to produce new and greater amounts of red blood cells. New red blood cells contain more hemoglobin, which increases the blood's oxygen-carrying capabilities, than old red blood cells.

Synthetic EPO has been developed for use in medical cases. Patients with leukemia (white blood cell cancer) or other cancers who undergo chemotherapy, radiation or a bone marrow transplant have severely decreased red blood cell counts. To help the body rebuild the count, they often receive EPO treatment, which benefits them tremendously Unfortunately, EPO has also been abused by athletes looking to cheat. There have been many cases in endurance sports, such as cycling and cross-country skiing, where athletes have injected themselves with EPO to boost their blood's oxygen-carrying capacity for training and competition. This practice is called blood doping. Some athletes have pushed the limits so far that their blood has become too thick, and heart attacks and premature deaths have been reported. The good news is that new testing techniques can identify synthetic EPO, so that doping with this hormone is now almost impossible.

There are "natural" ways to stimulate the body's EPO response. In altitude training, a controversial practice, athletes train at varying elevations above sea level to take advantage of the possible physiological effects on the human body. Exercise and living at high altitude may have a significant influence on oxygen transport and use. Some athletes and trainers believe that these metabolic and musculo-cardio-respiratory responses benefit athletes because they appear similar to the changes brought about by endurance training. Natives of high-altitude locations also display characteristics that may lead to enhanced endurance performance. The big problem with altitude training is that, because oxygen levels are lower at altitude, the absolute training intensity is also lower. Basically, athletes training at altitude feel like they are working harder than at sea level, but in fact they are working at lower intensities or speeds. Therefore, some aspects of the body can improve—for example, the blood's ability to carry oxygen. But other areas may actually get worse—muscle strength may decrease, for example.

The latest trend in altitude training is "live high/train low." In this scenario, athletes sleep at altitude or in altitude tents and then return to lower elevations to train. I had the opportunity of visiting a hotel in Finland which has rooms with special ventilation systems that lower the oxygen levels at night. Even though the occupants are actually at sea level, their bodies are fooled into adapting to altitude. More recent advances include tents that can be set up in a room. Air with oxygen levels lowered by nitrogen is pumped into the tent area. Spending time in the tent is thought to simulate altitude exposure.

Interestingly, levels of red blood cells appear to change in the weeks leading into a competition when athletes reduce their training volume, or "taper." Dr. Inigo Mujika, associate professor at the University of the Basque Country, reported that, during those weeks, blood parameters such as hemoglobin levels (the oxygen-carrying capacity of the red blood cells), hematocrit (the percentage of red blood cells in the blood) and red blood cell volume (the size of the red blood cells) were all increased.[3] Other

GREG'S HIGH-PERFORMANCE TIPS

REST HELPS YOUR BLOOD ADAPT

If you've been training hard for a few weeks or a few months, make sure to rest periodically to let your blood adapt. We suggest one recovery week every month for most people who are on an exercise routine. Before a job interview, sporting event or music performance, take it easy for two or three weeks. You can help your blood adapt by eating foods that are high in iron and vitamin C, which helps the body absorb iron.

researchers have found increases in reticulocyte counts (new red blood cells), suggesting an increased erythropoiesis (red blood cell production). These observations indicate that, when training loads are reduced, the body has extra energy to spend on building new and better red blood cells. This is excellent news for athletes. New red blood cells are more effective than older ones at transporting oxygen, and since hemoglobin is the molecule that binds oxygen, more hemoglobin means greater gas-carrying capacity. Interestingly, since hemoglobin is negatively charged, it also serves to buffer hydrogen ions, which are positively charged, and therefore increases the ability of the body to tolerate the lactic acid produced in high-intensity exercise.

Perhaps most importantly, Dr. Mujika found that athletes with the greatest improvement in post-taper red blood cell counts were those who improved the most in their sporting performance from pre- to post-taper. Improving red blood cell parameters is not just a random occurrence—it can be facilitated through nutrition. To provide the body with the building blocks it needs to make new red cells, I suggest athletes follow a diet high in iron during taper. Iron is used to make hemoglobin, so having enough in the system is critical to ensure the body can adapt. I also suggest eating foods that are high in vitamin C (such as citrus fruits) because it helps the body absorb iron.

A recent discovery related to exercise and genetics is that exercise can protect your DNA. In a recent study, researchers examined the DNA of young and old athletes and healthy control non-smokers for a total of four study groups. As expected, the researchers were able to demonstrate that the athletes had a slower resting heart rate, lower blood pressure and body-mass index, and a more favourable cholesterol profile. But the surprising finding was that the rate of accumulated damage to the DNA was much lower in the older athletes (average age, 51) than the older healthy non-athletes. In fact, the DNA of the older athletes was "younger" than that of the younger non-athlete participants. Researchers measured telomeres, which are the ends of the chromosomes that contain our DNA. Telomeres are like the caps on the end of your shoelaces that prevent the laces from fraying. (The scientists who discovered telomeres and how they work won the Nobel Prize in Physiology and Medicine in 2009). Telomeres control the number of times that a chromosome can divide when replicating itself throughout our lifetime. Cells naturally grow, divide to replicate themselves and then die off. Gradually through this replication process, telomeres shorten; when they become "critically short," the cell dies. On the whole-body level this may lead to ageing and a shortened lifespan. Scientists have shown that exercise activates an enzyme called telomerase, which protects telomeres and chromosomes and that this enzyme has an anti-ageing effect, especially on the cardiovascular system.

OXYGEN PATHWAY STEP 3: THE HEART

During an average human life, the heart will beat about three billion times. The heart is responsible for pumping blood through our bodies and, in the case of our pathway, must pump blood that has been oxygenated in the lungs out to our brain, organs and muscles through our circulatory system.

The heart is an organ made up of smooth muscle and serves to carry blood through the human body by using two different pumps, called ventricles. The blood comes to the heart from the peripheral organs low in oxygen. Blood coming from the upper part of the body is collected into the superior vena cava, while blood from the lower part of the body is collected into the inferior vena cava. The heart has two smaller chambers, called atria. These chambers ensure that the ventricles have a sufficient supply of blood for each contraction. The right atrium receives the deoxygenated blood directly from the vena cava and then pumps it through to the right ventricle, which then pumps it to the lungs. The left atrium receives the blood from the lungs (now oxygenated) and then pumps it into the left ventricle. The left ventricle then pumps the

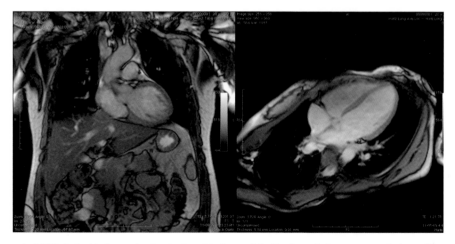

*An **MRI** of a healthy heart, showing the four chambers and the blood vessels that connect to the lungs. The image on the left is a view of the chest from the front. The image on the right is an overhead view.*

HOW TO USE HEART RATE TO CONTROL YOUR TRAINING

Heart rate is the key to gauging your aerobic intensity and building endurance. The most important investment you can make to monitor your aerobic training is a heart-rate monitor. If you don't have one, you can easily check your heart rate during exercise. Place your fingers between the trachea and the long muscle that runs next to your windpipe, feel for your pulse and then calculate your heart rate in beats per minute.

The next step is to calculate your maximum heart rate (HR$_{max}$). You can estimate your maximum heart rate by subtracting 0.85 times your age from 217:

$$Maximum\ heart\ rate = $$
$$217 - \underline{\quad}\ [0.85 \times your\ age] = $$
$$\underline{\quad}\ beats/minute\ (b/m)$$

This is just an estimate—the method will produce reasonable estimates in about 70% of the population. You can also have your maximum heart rate measured accurately by a physiologist or doctor. Consult your physician or trainer to have this test conducted if you want more accurate results. Once you know your maximum heart rate, you can calculate your aerobic cardiovascular training zones to help improve your endurance and health. I'll present my training zones in Chapter 7, Putting It All Together.

oxygenated blood to the rest of the body. Since the left ventricle has to pump blood through the entire body, it is larger and its muscle walls are thicker and stronger than those of the right ventricle, which has to pump blood only a short distance to the lungs.

The heart contracts in a constant rhythm that may speed up or slow down, depending on the need for blood (and oxygen) in the body. For example, if you start running, your leg muscles will need more oxygen to do the work. Therefore, your heart will have to pump more oxygen-carrying blood to those working muscles and will need to beat more rapidly to supply that blood. The beating of the heart is governed by an automatic electrical impulse generated by the sinus node, a small bundle of nerve fibres found in the wall of the right atrium near the opening of the superior vena cava. The sinus node generates an electrical charge, called an action potential. Once generated, it travels through the two atria and the two ventricles via the a-v node and the Purkinje fibres. The action potential causes the muscle walls of the heart to contract. The atria contract before the ventricles do—a sequence that allows the blood to be quickly pumped into the ventricles from the atria and then from the ventricles to the lungs and the rest of the body. The sinus node determines the rate at which the entire heart beats.

Heart rate is the term used to describe the number of times that the heart beats in one minute and is measured in beats per minute (b/m). When an adult is at rest, the normal heart rate can range from 40 b/m in a highly trained athlete to 70 b/m in an average person. Recent research has shown that your resting heart rate is associated with your lifespan—so if you have a high-resting heart rate, you are more likely to be affected by a chronic disease and have a shorter life.[4] People with low-resting heart rates have healthy cardiovascular systems, experience lower nervous system stress and are more likely to live longer.

For the purposes of the general population, the work of the heart, and by extension cardiovascular exercise intensity, can be roughly estimated by using the heart rate. To take your heart rate, place two fingers and apply light pressure between the trachea and the long muscle that runs up and down next to your windpipe to feel the pulse in your carotid artery. Then count the number of beats in 10 seconds (start counting at zero) and multiply by six to get the number of heartbeats in one minute, and thus the heart rate.

Resting heart rate is not the only factor to consider; the human heart has the capacity to increase its workload to fuel the body during times of physical demand, such as exercise. During intense exercise, the heart rate may increase up to 200 beats per minute, and occasionally even higher. The ventricles also fill up more to pump more blood with each beat—just like your lungs fill up more deeply when you are breathing harder. This ability to increase its workload helps the heart send blood, oxygen and nutrients to the body as needed through the peripheral circulatory system.

Carrying blood away from the heart to the muscles and organs, and then returning blood to the lungs and heart, are the vessels that make up the peripheral circulatory system. Vessels carrying blood away from the heart are called arteries, and those returning blood to the heart are called veins. As the arteries carry blood away from the heart, they branch into smaller and smaller vessels called arterioles. The arterioles also branch into smaller and smaller vessels until they are about

Arteries (red) take blood away from the heart and lungs. Veins (blue) collect blood from all over the body and return it to the heart. The colours are not just an artist's rendition; oxygenated blood really is red, while deoxygenated blood is blue/purple.

the width of one red blood cell. At this point, they are called capillaries. The capillaries are tiny vessels that allow for the transfer of oxygen and nutrients from the blood to muscles and organs and also allow blood to pick up the waste products and carbon dioxide from metabolism. As the blood begins to return to the heart, the capillaries connect to form increasingly larger vessels, called venules. The venules then merge into the larger veins.

Each of the body's vessels is made up of a tube composed of fibrous tissue. Smooth muscle cells surround the arterioles and the fibrous walls of the arteries and contract or relax to control air or blood flow. This enables the vessels of the peripheral circulatory system to regulate blood flow and alter the pattern of circulation throughout the body. For example, in exercise the vessels that supply blood to the stomach and intestines contract (thereby reducing blood flow in that area), and the vessels in and around the working muscles relax (thereby increasing blood flow and oxygen supply). A muscle's blood flow can increase up to 25 times during exercise. Veins have an additional feature that facilitates the return of blood to the heart, sometimes against the pull of gravity. They have valves that open when blood flows towards the heart (e.g., from the knee to the hip), and close when blood flows in the opposite direction. Blood can be pushed through veins in several ways: by smooth muscle that surrounds the veins, by contraction of large muscles near the veins, or, to a minor extent, by the pumping action of the heart.

Most people think that the activity of the heart is best measured by our heart rate, but in fact heart rate is only half the equation. The second part is stroke volume, which measures the amount of blood that's pumped out of the left ventricle each time the heart beats. Stroke volume is measured in millilitres. A typical stroke volume for a normal heart is about 70 millilitres of blood per beat. The product of stroke volume and heart rate is called the cardiac output. Cardiac output is measured in litres per minute (L/min) and can be described by the formula:

$$\text{Cardiac output} = \text{stroke volume} \times \text{heart rate}$$

Resting cardiac output in a healthy person is about 5 L/min. During maximum exercise, this rate can increase to 25 L/min, or even higher in trained athletes.

Blood pressure is an important measure of cardiac function. There are two components to blood pressure. The first, called diastole, is used to describe the pressure in the heart when the ventricles are relaxed and being filled with blood. Diastole is used as an indicator of peripheral blood pressure (the blood pressure in the body, outside the heart). The second component of blood pressure, called systole, is the pressure in the ventricles when they are contracting and pushing blood out into the body. The normal range of pressure in the atria during diastole is about 80 mmHg, and during systole about 120 mmHg. When you exercise, the heart muscle contracts more powerfully to push more blood to the body faster, so the systolic pressure increases at that time. The diastolic pressure, or the pressure when the heart is relaxed, should not change during exercise.

Exercise training can serve to increase stroke volume. Not surprisingly, many endurance athletes have an enlarged left ventricle, which is sometimes called "athlete's heart." Basically, when your heart pumps blood, the chambers in your heart eventually get better at pumping more blood with each beat—much like swimmers who pull more water with each stroke, or runners who leap farther with each stride as they train. Because the heart is so closely associated with life and death, any heart problem can be severe and often tragic. There are two main kinds of problems with the heart: the first stems from genetic defects that cause sudden cardiac death or other unexpected events in otherwise healthy people; the second includes the gradual onset of cardiovascular disease related to risk factors such as smoking, lack of activity or poor diet.

There is a long history of sudden cardiac death in athletes, dating back to the fifth century BC. The Greek herald Pheidippides ran 26 miles (41.8 kilometres) from Marathon to Athens to announce a Greek military victory, then died on the spot. There have been reports of this kind of catastrophic occurrence happening in modern times as well, with examples that include

GREG'S HIGH-PERFORMANCE TIPS
HEART SAFETY DURING EXERCISE

Fainting, seizures or dizziness is not normal during exercise, no matter how hard you are working. If you have experienced any of these symptoms, it is important to see a doctor to get cleared for safe participation. For more information, go to www.sads.ca

GREG'S HIGH-PERFORMANCE TIPS
STAIRWAY TO HEALTH

Adding stair climbing to your daily routine can be an easy way to fit in activity that can have a powerful impact on your body over time. As few as two flights of stairs climbed each day can lead to 6-lb weight loss over one year. A strong association exists between stair climbing and bone density in post-menopausal women. Stair-climbing programs can improve the amount of "good cholesterol" in the blood. Stair climbing also increases leg power and may play an important role in reducing the risk of injury from falls in the elderly.

Olympic gold-medal figure skater Sergei Grinkov in 1995, professional basketball player Reggie Lewis in 1993, college basketball player Hank Gathers in 1990 and Olympic volleyball champion Flo Hyman in 1986. More recently, Alem Techale, Ethiopia's 1500-metre star, collapsed and died during a training run in early 2005. Russian professional hockey player Alexei Cherepanov died while playing the game in 2008. While secondary prevention such as automatic external defibrillator (AED) deployment may save some athletes, as in the case of professional hockey player Jiri Fischer,[5] thus far survival has been less than expected among attempted resuscitations in intercollegiate athletes.[6] Sudden death due to heart attack remains the leading cause of non-traumatic death in athletes. Dr. Robert Hamilton at the Hospital for Sick Children in Toronto is currently suggesting that, before competing in any athletic activity, young athletes complete a three-step pre-participation screening procedure that includes (1) a personal history, (2) a family history and (3) a physical exam, including a 12-lead ECG.

OXYGEN PATHWAY STEP 4: THE MUSCLE AND MITOCHONDRIA

The final step in the oxygen transport pathway involves the muscles. The blood has finally carried oxygen from the environment through the lungs via the blood to where it is needed. Oxygen is absorbed into the muscle by diffusion from higher concentrations in the bloodstream to lower concentrations in the muscle. Once in the muscle, oxygen bonds with a molecule called myoglobin, which is very similar to hemoglobin except that it exists in muscle rather than blood. Myoglobin carries the oxygen to the mitochondria, which use oxygen to burn fuels such as carbohydrates and fats to produce energy for our muscles. (I will take a closer look at mitochondria in the following chapter.)

Cardiovascular Endurance Training

Fortunately, the cardiovascular system (the heart and blood vessels) responds to cardiovascular exercise such as walking or running and habitual physical activities such as housework or gardening. One only has to read the many stories of people who have come back from severe heart attacks and poor health to be marathon runners, century cyclists or triathletes to realize how much the body can change in response to consistent exercise. I can attest that, over my four-month bike ride through Africa, I was able to lose 33 pounds and went from being very unfit to competing in a semi-professional

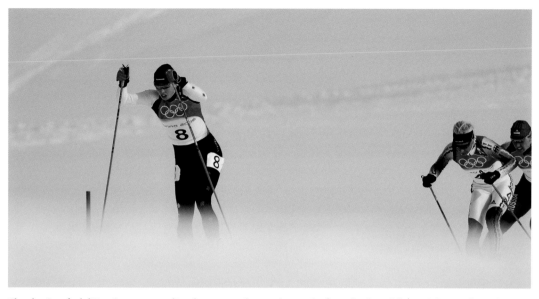

Chandra Crawford skiing. Cross-country skiers have tremendous cardiovascular fitness levels, with larger and more efficient hearts and lungs, a greater blood volume, and a higher concentration of red blood cells.

bike race from Montreal to Quebec City (300 kilometres) only seven months after starting training. Studies on patients who have had heart failure and then participated in a training program have shown improved maximal aerobic power (volume of oxygen that can be absorbed by the body or vo_{2max}) test results and increased arterial–venous O_2 difference. This means the skeletal muscles were able to absorb and use more oxygen. Other results show increased muscle blood flow, increased aerobic enzymes and more aerobic muscle fibres, all of which demonstrate just how powerful exercise is in improving the human body.

There are three primary types of aerobic exercise training that are really effective. (I'll describe them in detail in Chapter 7, Putting It All Together.) In this chapter, I'll show you, from a physiological perspective, how different kinds of training can help your oxygen transport system, your overall health and your ability to exercise for longer periods without getting tired .

Exercise and training for an improved aerobic cardiovascular system
Training your cardiovascular oxygen transport system is all about improving your aerobic endurance. You can train different aspects of your aerobic endurance ability through aerobic base training, high-intensity threshold training and recovery. Aerobic base training consists of

COMPOUNDS THAT CAN IMPROVE AEROBIC FUNCTION

Exercise training—even strength training—increases the amount of work done by the aerobic system. The body uses oxygen to fuel our muscles and to help them recover from anaerobic exercise and strength training. Aerobic respiration in our bodies produces free radicals (also called reactive oxygen species). Over time, our cells may become damaged by oxidation (similar to metal rusting when left out in the air for a long time). Antioxidant vitamins and minerals block the process of oxidation in the body by neutralizing free radicals. Antioxidant nutrients include vitamin E, vitamin C, beta-carotene, and the minerals selenium, manganese and zinc. I recommend taking an antioxidant supplement after your workouts. Here are a couple of examples of such supplements:

Glutathione. This supplement has positive effects on aerobic metabolism because it acts on the electron transport chain. Glutathione may help improve mitochondrial function. Consider this supplement if you are training for an endurance event such as a running race or a triathlon. Dietary sources include asparagus, broccoli, potatoes, walnuts, garlic, carrots, grapefruit, cauliflower, squash, okra, spinach, avocados and raw tomatoes. Freshness is key because the concentration of gluatathione decreases dramatically when foods are cooked, pasteurized or stored for a long time.

Coenzyme Q10. This substance has been used to treat mitochondrial muscle diseases. Dietary sources include meat, poultry and fish as well as soybean and canola oils.

increasing volumes of low-intensity exercise. This training sets the stage for the later development of your capacity to perform higher-intensity interval training. High-intensity threshold training involves performing exercise at the highest intensity a person can sustain for an extended period—usually 20 to 60 minutes, depending on the fitness level of the individual. Interval training is a highly effective technique that lets you alternate periods of exercise with periods of rest or low-intensity recovery exercise. Learning how to train in each zone is important to be sure that your training is efficient and effective, keeps you from becoming overtired, and is specific to your needs. Aerobic cardiovascular training should be performed at least three or four times a week for 15 to 60 minutes a session (or longer, if you are training for an event such as the triathlon or a running race). This training should be done throughout the year—actually, throughout your life. Always consult your doctor to make sure it's safe for you to start exercising.

Cardiovascular training has powerful effects on the entire oxygen transport system. From the lungs to the blood to the heart and right out to the muscles, the system adapts and improves itself to be able to handle the demands of exercise. The amazing thing is that not only does the body build itself up to handle exercise, but all the adaptations and changes help the body resist disease. Research has clearly shown that cardiovascular exercise reduces the incidence of diabetes, heart disease, cancer and many other diseases. Here's a figure that shows the improvements in the oxygen transport system that result from cardiovascular training. Imagine if a drug were developed that could do all that! It would be front-page news across the world. Well, we have that power. We just have to commit to doing some form of exercise consistently over an extended period. In the following chapters, I will talk about other systems in the body and how they are pushed to the limit during extreme activities. I'll also add to the above training plan when we talk about muscles in Chapter 2 and nerves Chapter 3. In Chapter 6, I'll show you how to speed your recovery from exercise so you can live and work at a higher level all the time. In Chapter 7, I'll show you several examples of week plans that incorporate more complex training.

THE OXYGEN PATHWAY

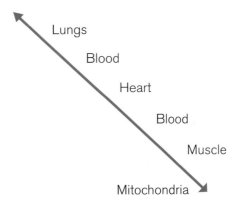

With exercise training, each step of the pathway adapts. The lungs increase in volume, more red blood cells are produced that carry more hemoglobin, and the heart increases in volume. The muscle changes fibre types to meet the demands of training and more mitochondria are produced.

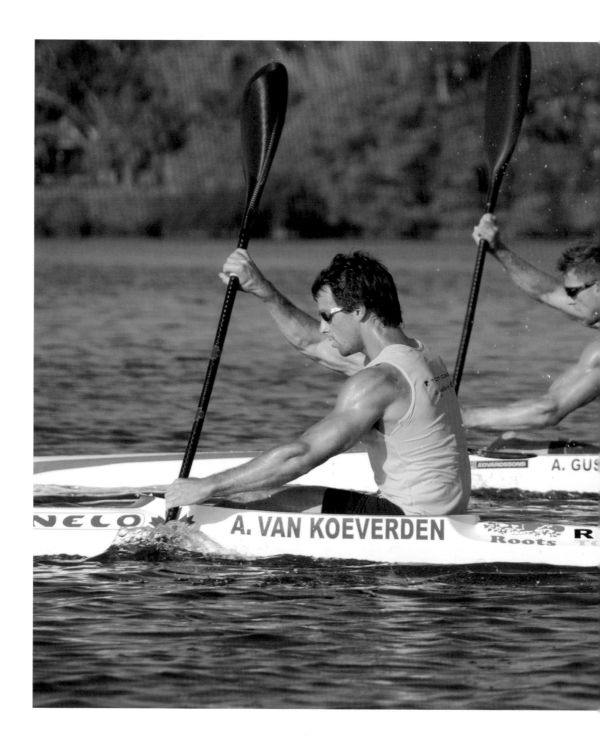

POWERING HUMAN MOVEMENT

THE MUSCULOSKELETAL SYSTEM

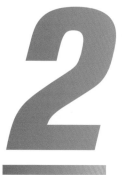

Muscles are extraordinary structures. They have the ability to change themselves to meet the demands that you impose on them. Running for the bus or lifting objects over your head gets easier if you do these things every day because your muscles actually change and adapt. The ancient Greeks knew this, and their history includes the story of Milo of Croton, who was a six-time Olympic champion in wrestling. It is said that he trained by lifting a bull over his head, starting when it was a calf and continuing every day until it was full grown. As the bull grew, so did Milo of Croton's strength, or so the story goes. There may be some truth to this story. Modern Olympians give us an idea of just how much our muscles can adapt, changing in response to training for endurance events such as the marathon, or sprint events such as the 100-metre dash. We can even create the characteristic of pure strength as exhibited in weightlifting, or the pure power we see in the explosive jumps that basketball players use to dunk a ball. Even more amazing are athletes who can train their muscles for both endurance and strength, such as tennis players who compete for hours but have to call on explosive power when they hit shots.

Throughout history, human beings have pushed the limits of what we consider possible. Even when we think we can't possibly get faster, higher or stronger, an athlete comes along and defies our expectations, establishing new world records. Think of the four-minute mile (1.6 kilometres) or the 10-second 100-metre dash. Both were thought impossible to break. Now they're performed routinely. Pushing the limits is a part of sport—actually, it's part of being human. But what does pushing the limit mean? What limits us? When we run up a flight of stairs, we feel like our muscles and lungs are burning. When we work all day and we get tired, our bodies and our brains become fatigued. How does this happen? Scientists are still debating why the body gets tired, but the question of why we experience fatigue hasn't been answered. We can gain some insight, however, by looking closely at the muscles. I'll show you how these muscles are built and how they work.

We have more than 300 muscles in our bodies. Together, they make up about 35% and 45% of the body mass in women and men, respectively.[7] Muscles support most of our major life functions: our breathing, physical movement and digestion, and the pumping of life-sustaining blood throughout the body. When you think of muscle, you probably think of the main kind of muscle—skeletal muscle, which makes up the muscles we use to voluntarily control movement. But there are other kinds of muscles as well. We have a special type of muscle called smooth muscle, which lines the walls of our blood vessels, the iris of the eyes and the walls of the digestive tract (stomach and intestines). This type of muscle, which is controlled unconsciously, regulates the flow of blood through the blood vessels, changes the size of the iris in our eyes to control how much light hits the retina, breaks down food in the stomach and helps move partially digested food through the intestines. Smooth muscle is very fatigue-resistant. The heart is a specialized muscle, called a cardiac muscle, which is extremely powerful and also highly resistant to fatigue—a good thing, because you wouldn't want your heart to get tired.

MUSCLE STRUCTURE

Both muscles and tendons are critical to movement. When you decide to move, your brain sends signals down the spinal cord to nerves connected to the body of the muscle. When the electrical signal from the brain reaches the muscle, special proteins called neurotransmitters are released into the space between the nerve and the muscle. These neurotransmitters carry the signal to contract from the nerve to the muscles, and when they arrive at the surface of the muscle they connect to receptors.

These receptors then change their structure, resulting in a cascade of chemical events in the muscle that leads to contraction. The muscle shortens and pulls on the tendons that are attached to bones, making the bones move. Tendons also contain stretch receptors that help prevent sudden, sharp over-stretching of the muscle to protect it from tearing. So, although movement seems simple, it is a complicated process involving the brain, the spinal cord, electricity, neuro-chemicals, muscles, tendons and bones. Think about that

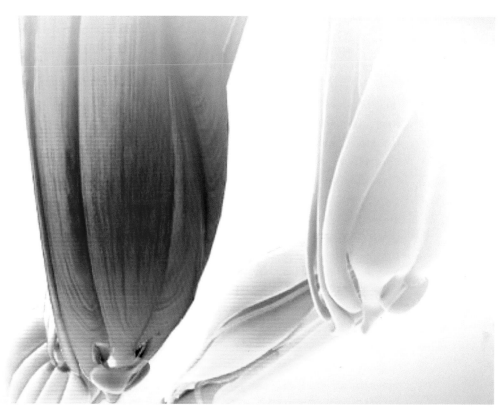

Skeletal muscles are actually made up of bundles of fibres bound together by connective tissue. They are usually connected to bones by special collagen fibres called tendons.

the next time you perform the simple movement of reaching for a glass of water. And watch in amazement when people perform incredibly complicated movements at speed, like table tennis players who can return a tiny ball flying at them at high velocity. It's also easy to understand how muscles can become dysfunctional in diseases such as muscular dystrophy.

MUSCLE CONTRACTION

As I mentioned, muscles are actually made up of smaller cylindrical cells called muscle fibres. Many muscle fibres are bundled together to make up a particular muscle. Muscle fibres are about 1/10 of a millimetre thick, but they can be very long. For example, the muscle fibres in the biceps can be as long as 15 centimetres. Fibres are built for contraction and contain complex structures and chemicals that produce energy from the foods we eat. The fibres themselves are actually made up of smaller structures called myofilaments. The contractile apparatus in each myofilament is made up of proteins called actin and myosin.

We are not absolutely sure how muscles contract, but our best guess right now involves the sliding filament theory. During the contraction of a muscle, it is the thin actin filaments sliding over the thick myosin filaments that cause a shortening of the muscle to create movement. When a signal to contract reaches the muscle, the actin proteins link up with the myosin's heavy chain proteins. This linkage allows the actin filaments to slide relative to the myosin chains, shortening the muscle and creating a contraction. To help you visualize this process, think of a rowboat with many rowers. The oars drop into and pull on the water to move the boat forward. Then they lift out of the water, move backward and drop into the water again for the next stroke. A similar process occurs in the muscle to shorten the muscle fibres, create a contraction and produce movement.

MUSCLE FIBRE TYPES

Not every type of movement is of the cardio endurance type just mentioned. Of course we can run, but we can also sprint, jump and lift. These explosive activities place different demands on our muscles. To meet these demands, different muscle fibre types have evolved. We have several kinds of muscle fibres, each with different characteristics. Skeletal muscle is composed of a mixture of two contractile fibre types: slow twitch and fast twitch. Each of the fibre types can be described by the main metabolic pathway that provides its energy. Slow-twitch fibres (also known as type I) are called oxidative. Fast-twitch fibres are subdivided into two types: fast-twitch oxidative-glycolytic (type IIa), and fast-twitch glycolytic (type IIb).

The slow-twitch fibres are red, and the fast-twitch fibres are white. The differences in colour are due to the increased levels of iron in the former. Blood is red because it has iron in the hemoglobin that carries oxygen. Slow-twitch muscle fibres have iron in myoglobin (the muscles' hemoglobin molecule) because they need lots of oxygen for aerobic metabolism. You would use your slow-twitch fibres for activities of daily living (e.g., walking) as well as for power-endurance exercise (e.g., running). You can also see that slow-twitch fibres are thin, and fast-twitch fibres are thicker. Fast-twitch fibres have more contractile proteins, giving these fibres a greater cross-sectional area. Fast-twitch fibres are used for higher-intensity activities like lifting, jumping and throwing.

Slow-Twitch Oxidative Fibres (Type I)

Slow-twitch fibres are just that—slow. They are used for the low-intensity activities of daily living, such as walking or doing tasks around the house. They are also used for long-duration activities—which require sustained, low-intensity energy outputs—including hiking, low-intensity cycling and jogging. If you undergo endurance training for a length of time, slow-twitch muscles adapt and become more efficient to be able to supply enough energy for longer-duration events such as marathons or mountain climbing. To fuel long-duration activities, slow-twitch muscles have a high concentration of organelles called mitochondria. These are the energy factories of the cell, producing energy by using oxygen to break down foods.

Mitochondria are very efficient, but the energy is produced at a relatively slower rate. In slow-twitch–type muscle fibres, oxygen is a key molecule, and therefore capillaries grow next to the fibres to supply them with the oxygen they need to fuel energy production. Thus, slow-twitch muscles have a low-power output but are quite fatigue-resistant.

Fast-Twitch Fibres (Types IIa and IIb)

Interestingly, muscles have evolved in a balanced way so that fast-twitch fibres function in an almost opposite manner to slow-twitch ones. They provide high-power outputs but fatigue more quickly. Fast-twitch oxidative fibres (type IIa) are a mix of both fast and slow twitch—they have a moderate power-producing capability and some fatigue resistance. These are the primary movers for events that last from 1 to 3 minutes—you use them when sprinting for a bus or running up a flight of stairs. Pure fast-twitch glycolytic fibres (type IIb) break down sugars such as glucose for

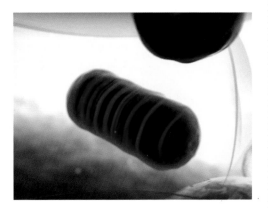

energy, and they don't need oxygen to produce energy. That's why they're sometimes called anaerobic, which means "without oxygen." Fast-twitch glycolytic fibres are used for explosive-type activities that involve very high power—jumping or short sprints, for example. They fatigue in as little as 10 seconds but produce huge amounts of power. Another extraordinary quality of muscles is that fast-twitch fibres can adapt to being more efficient oxidatively or glycolytically, depending on the type of training you do.

Most of the large muscles of the body have about even percentages of slow- and fast-twitch fibres, so they can perform both long duration and short powerful movements. Some muscles, like the gastrocnemius (the big muscle of your calf), are generally composed of about 60% slow-twitch fibres. This makes sense because the gastrocnemius is a primary muscle for walking, meaning we can go a long way without getting tired. But this muscle is also important for running and jumping, so it has about 40% fast-twitch fibres. Some elite athletes have slightly higher percentages of certain fibre types in muscles, simply by the luck of genetics—picking the right parents! It's a big advantage if you're a sprinter and have a slightly higher concentration of fast-twitch fibres in muscles used for running, or if you're an endurance athlete and have a higher concentration of slow-twitch fibres in muscles used for that activity.

Fibre Types and Energy

To generate movement, muscles need to contract. And to contract, they need energy—*lots* of energy. Each muscle fibre type has a matching energy production system that's used to provide the muscle cell with energy. Slow-

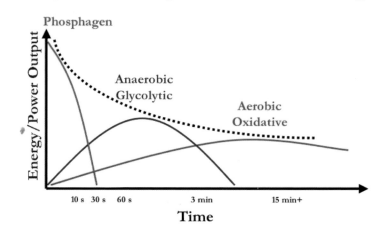

The body has three chemical systems to produce energy for muscle contractions.

twitch oxidative fibres rely mostly on the aerobic oxidative system, helping you run that marathon or do your triathlon. Fast-twitch oxidative fibres rely on a combination of the aerobic and anaerobic glycolytic systems, which provide for activities like sprinting. And fast-twitch glycolytic fibres rely mostly on the anaerobic system and the high-energy phosphate system to help fuel such high-intensity movements as taking a jump shot during a basketball game or lifting weights in the gym.

How Muscle Fibre Types Work Together to Create Performance

At this point, things start to get a bit complicated. Your muscles are made up of a combination of various fibre types. Even within fibres, the three different energy systems (aerobic, anaerobic and high-energy phosphate) can all contribute to fuelling movement at the same time. The key to understanding these combinations is to recall the main job of each fibre type and each energy system, and to remember that the different fibres and energy systems work together to help your body perform activities.

If you look at a mixed sport like the 1500-metre run—the famous mile—you can see how all the fibres and energy systems work together. The mile takes about four minutes for a world-class runner. At the beginning of the race, the athletes line up at the start line and get ready to run. As soon as the gun goes off, they accelerate up to race speed as quickly as possible. To do this, they recruit their fast-twitch fibres, because they react quickly, have high-power output and contract strongly to accelerate the body from rest to race speed. To fuel the fast-twitch fibres, the high-energy

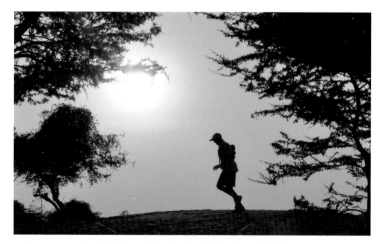

Ferg Hawke running through the Thar desert in India.

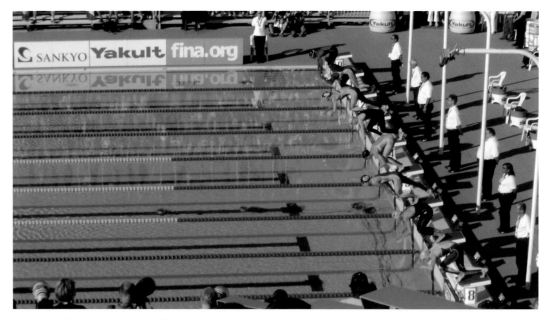

A start at world swimming championships. Notice the two American swimmers in the blue and grey suits have the fastest starts. Nervous-system training plays a key role in reaction time in speeding events.

phosphate system is activated immediately to provide ATP (adenosine triphosphate, which is stored in the muscle) for muscle contraction. Stored ATP provides enough energy for 8 to 10 seconds. The breakdown products of the high-energy phosphate system (the "exhaust," so to speak—in this case, adenosine di-phosphate) activates the anaerobic glycolytic system, which breaks down sugars to produce energy for muscle contraction at the very beginning of the race. This system can provide energy for only about 1 to 3 minutes, when the athlete is exercising at maximum capacity.

The "exhaust" of the anaerobic glycolytic system is a substance called lactic acid. Lactic acid is involved in muscle fatigue, so athletes have to reduce their speed to a sustainable level if they want to finish the four-minute event. This sustainable level is the rate at which energy can be provided by the aerobic system operating in the mitochondria that fuel the fast-twitch oxidative fibres and the slow-twitch fibres. So from just a few seconds into the race, right through to when the athletes start their finishing kick or sprint to the line, their muscles rely primarily on type IIa and type I fibres. Close to the end of the race, the athletes will estimate the point at which they can increase their speed above their sustainable level (also called their anaerobic threshold), re-engage their type IIa and

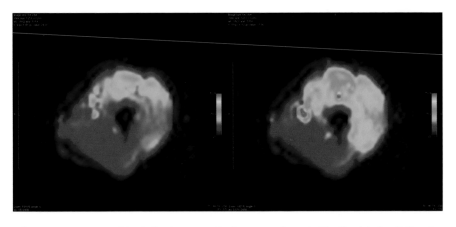

*A functional **MRI** image of the thigh. The green and red sections indicate the blood levels before (left) and after (right) exercise.*

IIb fibres and sprint to the line. Hopefully, they have estimated correctly, because these fibres exhaust their energy supplies rapidly. If an athlete miscalculates, he or she may end up fatiguing too early or waiting too long to begin the final sprint, and either way will likely lose the race. As you can see, even though the mile is just a four-minute event, it relies on all muscle fibre types and all energy systems.

MUSCLES AND BLOOD FLOW

To deliver nutrients to each bundle of muscle fibres, we have tiny blood vessels called capillaries. Capillaries also remove waste products. Amazingly, when you do cardiovascular endurance training, as described in Chapter 1, you can grow more capillaries to increase the amount of blood, oxygen and nutrients that can be delivered to the muscle and organs, including the heart. In contrast, lack of exercise results in decreased capillarization, or even blockages in the blood vessels, stopping blood from flowing to the tissues. That's what happens in a heart attack, where blood flow to a section of heart muscle stops, or in a stroke, where blood flow to a part of the brain is blocked. This increase in the number of capillaries is one way exercise training protects the heart and brain from cardiovascular disease. There

GREG'S HIGH-PERFORMANCE TIPS

USE CAFFEINE AS A TOOL, NOT A CRUTCH

Caffeine is effective for enhancing performance in athletes in low-to-moderate dosages (3 to 6 mg/ kg). *Use it as a tool, not a crutch.* It's most effective 30 minutes before a presentation, workout or other performance event.

are many avenues for blood and, therefore, oxygen delivery, to most tissues, including muscles, bones, the liver and even the brain.

As you can see in the functional MRI graphic above, quadriceps extensions caused increased blood flow through the tissues (light green areas) and also increased blood flow through veins and arteries (red areas). This concept (that blood flow increases with exercise) is pretty simple, but it is still very cool to see it happening when you take images. The MRI technique is totally non-invasive and, unlike a CAT scan or an X-ray, requires no radiation. So it has great potential to help assess muscle function in a number of diseases, including peripheral vascular disease.

MUSCLES AND FATIGUE

Lactic acid contributes to the fatigue process. If you've recently heard that this statement isn't true—and that lactic acid is in fact a fuel for muscle—please read on. Lactic acid is a fuel for muscle. But it does play a role in fatigue. Let's consider a sprint event—the 100-metre butterfly (100-metre fly) in swimming. It's a great event to analyze because the butterfly is a difficult stroke for most people. It's also the event that Michael Phelps won by 0.01 seconds in the 2008 Olympics, on his way to winning eight gold medals. The 100-metre fly takes very little time—about 50 seconds to complete if you're swimming at the Olympics—and the energy output is very high. Muscles are stimulated to contract with great force as quickly as possible, while the brain adjusts the motor patterns to ensure the athlete sustains the required technique.

Since the muscle power and energy consumption are high, the brain recruits all fibre types (I, IIa and IIb) to help move the athlete through the water. Within the muscle itself, both the fast-twitch oxidative and glycolytic fibres break down stored sugars for energy into a form of sugar called glycogen. Glycogen is broken down into glucose, and then, through a series of steps, into a substance called pyruvate. This process of breaking down sugars in the muscle is called glycolysis, which is why the fast-twitch fibre energy system is termed the anaerobic glycolytic system. Glycolysis does not require oxygen to function, and produces energy in the form of ATP very quickly. This ATP is used to fuel muscle contraction during the butterfly stroke. But there's a problem, and anyone who has tried to swim 100 metres of butterfly—even Michael Phelps—has experienced it. You've probably experienced it, too, when you run up stairs or sprint to catch a bus.

Because of the high muscle-energy demand, glucose is broken down faster than it can be processed in the mitochondria. This causes the accumulation of a substance called lactic acid. It's this acid that causes a burning sensation in our muscles and makes it hard to keep working at the same intensity. Lactic acid breaks apart into a lactate molecule and a hydrogen ion. The hydrogen ion—not the lactate—increases acidity and disrupts the metabolism of the muscle cell. Nerve fibres sense the acid buildup in the muscles and let the brain know there are metabolic problems in them. The lactate is stored until the intensity of the exercise decreases. It is then converted back into pyruvate and processed in the mitochondria, or reconverted back into glucose or glycogen for storage (this process is called gluconeogenesis). So lactic acid is both a fuel (the lactate part) *and* a fatigue agent (the acid part).

For an athlete to finish the 100-metre swim, one of two things must happen. First, the athlete must slow down and work aerobically to process fuels through the mitochondria. Second, as shown by Michael Phelps, the athlete is so well trained that he is able to use his aerobic system at such a high rate that not much lactic acid is accumulated—or, if it does accumulate, the athlete is able to maintain speed and fight through the mental and physical pain of this buildup to the end of the race.

Let's explore this fatigue process in a bit more detail. Hydrogen ions make fluids acidic. High acidity is a physiological challenge for muscle cells because the enzymes they employ to break down foods into useable energy sources work only within a narrow range of acidity. When the fluids inside muscle cells become acidic, the enzymes don't work very well and the creation of new energy is slowed. This is muscle fatigue. Think about running up a flight of stairs and your muscles starting to burn. If you go up the next flight as fast as you can, you probably start to feel your legs tighten up and you slow down. You're actually feeling your muscles' acidity change.

The excess hydrogen ions also create problems in the contractile apparatus of the muscle proteins. It is thought that increased levels of hydrogen ions disrupt the ability of actin and myosin proteins to link up, and therefore contraction of the muscle becomes difficult.

You can see this fatigue happen quite often in sports, where athletes push themselves to the limit in races that last from 1 to 6 minutes. On the third day of the 2010 Olympics in Vancouver, Sven Kramer from the Netherlands won a gold medal in the 5000-metre track speed-skating event. He showed determination and aggressiveness right from the start of the 6:14-minute race, and as a result we saw some interesting biomechanics and physiology. Athletes and coaches measure great technique as "distance per stride." Simply put, athletes apply force against the water, ground or ice,

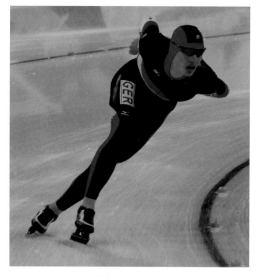

Speed skating is incredibly demanding technically and physiologically. The skater's muscles have to work very hard to drive the skater forward against the ice. To reduce wind drag, the core and back muscles have to stabilize the skater's upper body parallel to the ice. And to supply enough oxygen to the working muscles, the skater has to breathe up to 200 litres of air, per minute, in and out of the lungs. At this intensity, type IIa and IIb glycolytic muscle fibres are activated and lactic acid begins to accumulate.

and the power of that force minus the resistive forces is the efficiency of their movement, which dictates how far they travel. The challenge is to keep that distance per stride and then increase the number of strides per minute to maximize speed. At the start of the race, Sven Kramer was skating fast and also holding great distance per stride. This performance was fine as long as he kept fatigue at bay, which he could not do because of his aggressiveness at the start of the race. As the fatigue factors accumulated in his body, his technique gradually deteriorated. His strides became shorter, and his body position became more vertical. As soon as skaters become too tired to hold the proper body position with the torso as parallel to the ice as possible, wind resistance increases dramatically. This effect compounds the fatigue even further because it becomes increasingly difficult to keep moving forward at the speed required. The challenge is to maintain technique despite the physiological fatigue. We were able to see the fatiguing effects of lactic acid accumulation near the end of the race, when Kramer's face was a mask of agony and he had to use his hands to push his legs for the last few strides across the finish line. In this case, the pain was worth the gain—he won a gold medal.

Watching events such as swimming and speed skating, where athletes push themselves into the anaerobic metabolism zone that produces lactic acid, is especially interesting when you consider the adaptations the body has developed to handle the metabolic by-products of intense exercise. Dr. Arend Bonen from the University of Guelph, a former competitive swimmer himself, has published an interesting review paper on the specialized proteins that reside on the surface of muscle cells, called monocarboxylate transporters.[8] These transporters work to shuttle lactic acid out of the type II fast-twitch muscle fibres into the blood, where lactate and hydrogen ions are transported to type I slow-twitch muscle fibres that have lots of mitochondria that can process the lactate and use it as fuel. Think of them as microscopic "taxis" that move lactate around the muscle fibres as needed. The transporters on

MUSCLE ADAPTATIONS TO RESTING BEFORE COMPETITION

Several studies have examined the effects of tapering (reducing training loads before competition) on muscle contractile properties and their ability to produce power. By resting during the taper phase, muscles actually increase their ability to produce power. This improvement appears somewhat counterintuitive, but the effects are significant. It seems that taper results in changes to type II fibres more than type I. Researchers have shown that the actual contractile properties of the muscle fibres change and that type II fibres increase in size, strength, velocity and power.[9] New contractile actin and myosin proteins are produced, muscle fibres get thicker and stronger, and improvements in whole body strength and power result.

To facilitate these changes and ensure athletes get the rest they need, I recommend decreasing or even stopping resistance training ("strength" training) for 10–15 days before an event. This taper period allows adequate time for muscles to rebuild and regenerate before the start of competition. It's also advisable to avoid eccentric muscle contractions (applying tension while lengthening the muscle) during taper, because this type of muscle stress can cause micro-tears that take additional time to repair. The amazing fact here is that the time during the training year when the muscle adapts the fastest appears to be when athletes are training the least.

the surface of type II fibres that get lactic acid out of the muscle cell are different from those on the surface of the type I fibres that pull lactic acid into the slow-twitch muscle fibres. It's an amazing adaptation the body has evolved to create a protein that clears waste products from one type of muscle cell and takes it to a different type, where it can be recycled into stored fuel or immediate energy. It's the muscles' own version of green energy.

Extreme Fatigue: Hitting the Wall

A fascinating physiological phenomenon is that of marathon runners "hitting the wall" and becoming severely fatigued near the end of the 26-mile (41.8 kilometre) race. Well, it may be fascinating for me; probably not so much for the runners experiencing it at the time. The actual physiological mechanism that explains why this phenomenon happens is still highly debated, but there are some likely candidates. Lactic acid accumulation is associated with muscle fatigue, but only in short, high-intensity activities such as sprinting. Since the marathon is a 2- to 3-hour-long event (perhaps longer if you're a sub-elite runner), it's unlikely that the intensities are high enough for lactic acid to accumulate to cause muscle fatigue. One possibility is that the internal temperature of the body rises and may be magnified if the athlete becomes dehydrated and stops sweating. Another is that the majority of the stored fuels (e.g., muscle glycogen) have been used up, and as a result blood glucose may decrease. Some researchers think that the brain monitors the levels of these fuels in our bodies, and if the levels of substances such as glucose decrease to a dangerous level, then the brain shuts down muscle activity by creating the sensation of muscle fatigue. This theory is known as the "central governor" theory of fatigue. It's important to note that it's just a theory, and a relatively new one at that, so more research is needed.

Extreme Fatigue: Muscle Damage

Running out of energy and overheating are not the only challenges for the muscles during exercise and sport. Sometimes extreme forces are enough to cause micro-damage to the muscle fibres. You can see the effects of these huge forces in many sports. One of the reasons I love the Winter Olympics so much is that they are, for the most part, performed on ice and snow, and that means more speed and greater height. It also means greater risk and more micro-damage to muscle cells. In no sport is this more relevant than alpine skiing. Studying alpine skiing is so much fun for me as a scientist because it allows me to look at the performance of the human body at the outside limit of its abilities. Alpine skiers have to push the envelope of their capabilities just to compete, let alone have any chance of winning. Think about these elements:

- ▸ often more than a kilometre of vertical drop
- ▸ speeds of more than 130 kilometres an hour
- ▸ a course that's made up mostly of ice
- ▸ skis with edges as sharp as razor blades

That's just the beginning. To win, you have to go as fast as you can while staying in control. Successful skiers can bring themselves right to the edge and hold themselves there for the entire two minutes of the race. A bunch of other factors make the performances of downhill skiers even more amazing. The first is what happens during all the turns. Basically, type II fast-twitch muscles in the legs, glutes and back contract simultaneously as the skier enters the turn to fight against their inertia in one direction. This contraction helps to change direction around the turn.

The reason this effort is so hard on the body is that, while the muscles are contracting, the skier is also being loaded with extra forces and the muscle myofibrils can get torn more easily. This is called an eccentric

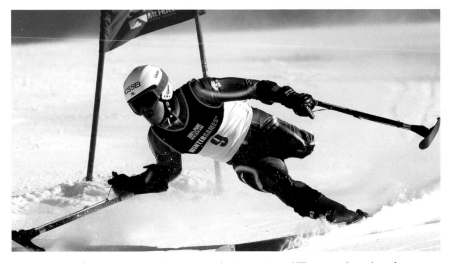

Hiraku Misawa of Japan competes in the Super G in the Winter Games NZ in 2011. Alpine skiers face significant challenges, including altitude, cold and speeds of up to 130 kilometres per hour.

contraction—a lengthening of the muscles while they are under load. These micro-tears are why we get sore when we lift weights or do a lot of unaccustomed exercise. Skiers train for years to be able not only to handle this physical stress, but also to push the body as hard as they can when it matters the most. In the slalom events, this means up to 65 turns (women) or 75 turns (men) in one race.

The other factor affecting the muscles in alpine skiing is the difficulty of racing in the cold. Alpine skiers often race in conditions well below freezing. Cold causes the body to try to preserve its heat, and it does so by shifting blood flow from the skin and muscles into the internal organs in the chest and belly. The effect of this shift is that the skiers feel sluggish because of the decreased blood flow to the arms and legs. Don't be surprised to see skiers jumping around and hitting their arms and legs, trying to keep warm and reactivate their circulatory systems right before they start. Maybe you've done this yourself when you're on the slopes.

Environmental conditions such as cold and heat can put enormous stress on the human body. When we exercise, we break down sugars and fats in the muscles to produce energy. This action releases heat. The body works well only within a certain temperature range and is highly adapted to stay in that range. Skiing in the cold is an example of such adaptation. The main physiological response to the cold is that the body has to produce more heat to keep the core body temperature regulated. Wind can exacerbate the

Shivering is a survival mechanism that the body uses to protect itself from colder temperatures. Most systems in the body work only within a narrow temperature range. When the body's temperature drops, the body signals the muscles to start contracting in short, fast bursts—hence, we shiver. These muscle contractions increase energy metabolism in the muscle cell, burn fuel and produce heat. This is the body's way of surviving in the short term, when its core temperature is too low. If you're ever out in the cold and find yourself shivering, that means it's time to go somewhere to get warm, fast.

problem by increasing the rate at which heat is removed from the body, thus increasing the heat production requirements. During exercise in the cold, the body shifts toward carbohydrate metabolism for energy, so eating foods high in complex carbohydrates will allow the body to produce energy more easily. Complex carbohydrates are found in whole-wheat products, so whole-wheat bread or bagels would be good options. When the body is exposed to the cold it will try to protect the more important systems (our internal organs) at the expense of the extremities (the hands and feet). Simply put, the body decreases the amount of blood that flows to the skin and the hands. Less blood flow means less fine-muscle control and coordination. The cold has a diuretic effect (increased urination), so hydration is as much of an issue in the cold as it is in the heat. When you consider all these physiological effects, the performances of winter sport athletes can be even more amazing to behold.

At the other end of the spectrum of environmental conditions is exercising in the heat. This can be extremely problematic, because it becomes difficult for the body to release heat when the environment is as hot as or hotter than the body itself. The body takes heat away from the exercising muscles through the blood. Blood passing through the muscles picks up the heat and follows the circulatory pathway to the veins on the way back to the heart. To allow the heat to escape, blood vessels in the skin open up, and blood is passed through the skin on its way back to the heart. Heat is transferred from the blood to the skin and to water in the sweat glands. This water passes up to the surface of the skin as sweat, and when the water evaporates off the skin, heat is pulled from the body and into the surrounding air. Heat management, sweating and hydration are the primary challenges in sports such as beach volleyball and other activities played outside in the heat.

If there is no sweating, the situation can become very dangerous. The body now has no means to cool itself, and its temperature will rise to dangerous levels. Most body functions operate only within a very narrow temperature range, so functions shut down when that range is exceeded. This condition is called heat exhaustion and (when more serious) heatstroke, and can result in unconsciousness or worse. The body must be cooled immediately to prevent adverse events.

I had my own experience with exercise in the heat and heat exhaustion. As I was cycling out of Khartoum, Sudan, during the Tour D'Afrique, the temperature was 50°C (120°F). To add to my wonderful first day of riding through the desert, I missed seeing the turnoff into our camp, and went an extra 50 kilometres, reaching a total of 170 kilometres for my first day of riding. The next day I drank 16 litres of water during the eight hours of cycling, and did not urinate once. I was covered in salt from all the evaporated sweat that came off my body during the day. About two-thirds of the way into the 120-kilometre day, I began to feel truly awful and almost started hallucinating. My muscles actually stopped and refused to pedal. I've done some pretty tough sporting events, and I swam competitively at a reasonably high level, so I know how to push myself. But there was nothing I could do to move my bike forward. My friend Andrew Griffin, who was on the trip with me and who is in the *Guinness Book of World Records* for the fastest human-powered crossing of Africa, pulled up next to me while I was resting on the side of the gravel trail. He said that I looked positively grey and that we should probably stop cycling for the day. We rested for an hour under the only tree we could find, and eventually I cooled off enough to be able to function again. In hindsight, it was clear that I was well on my way to heat exhaustion and possibly even heatstroke. This was embarrassing, given that I had just finished a PhD in exercise physiology. This experience was a major life learning point for me—it's not just knowledge that counts, but knowing how to apply and manage your knowledge in the real world. I didn't get heat exhaustion again on that trip.

Fortunately, we can use our knowledge of physiology and heat transfer to help us perform better, or just to exercise comfortably in the environment. For example, when you're exercising, or just out in the cold, wear darker-coloured clothing; it helps to absorb heat and to keep you warmer. The opposite holds true in warm weather. Lighter-coloured clothing reflects light and heat away from the body and keeps you cooler (although the New Zealand All Blacks Rugby team has tested this idea and denies that dark clothing has a negative effect). Hats are critical in both conditions. Imagine the difference in your performance if, on a hot day, you were to play golf wearing a black hat, which absorbs light and heat, vs. a white one, which reflects heat away from the head. New fabrics that "wick" sweat away from the skin are also excellent for keeping you cool in hot conditions. This helps

RUNNING BAREFOOT VS. RUNNING WEARING SHOES... WHAT DOES THE RESEARCH SAY?

The recent popularity of running barefoot has taken many people by surprise and ignited quite a debate in both running circles and the research community. Although some people think that barefoot running is a new phenomenon, in reality the use of padded and supported running shoes is a recent development—as recent as the 1970s. So, in fact, we may be getting back to basics and the way the foot evolved.

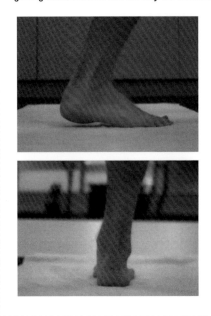

The proponents of barefoot running suggest that when people run barefoot, the tendency is to actually land on the ball of the foot and on the mid-foot. When this happens, the arch of the foot, not the heel bone, absorbs the impact, and as a result the impact forces are not transferred up the body but are absorbed by the muscles of the foot and lower leg. Supporters of the barefoot-running philosophy argue that it is healthier for the feet and reduces the risk of chronic injuries—although the research is not conclusive either way. But it's interesting, given that studies suggest that at least 30% of runners get injured every year, and many of these injuries stem from problems that arise in the foot or lower leg. On my website (http://www.drgregwells.com/wells-blog/2010/8/8/running-barefoot-vs-with-shoes-what-does-the-research-say.html), you can check out this video of a colleague running barefoot that was taken from the side, and you can see that in fact the heel never touches the ground. Proponents argue that this is why barefoot running is healthier than running with shoes.

maintain the ability of the skin to dissipate heat through sweat. Likewise, in cold weather, wicking clothing keeps the skin dry, and thus less heat is drawn away from it. In fact, hypothermia, or low body temperature, is often caused by exercising in the cold. But it's not during the exercise phase that hypothermia happens, because at that stage the body is producing lots of heat in the working muscles. Hypothermia occurs when the person stops exercising but is still sweating. So the body is no longer producing heat, but the sweating process remains active—pulling heat from the body through the skin and wet clothing, drawing the body temperature down.

WHAT HAPPENS WHEN... MUSCLES DON'T WORK

Muscles are not only critical for movement, exercise and sports; they also play a role in health. Physical activity, fitness and health outcomes are strongly

Some runners have achieved great success using this technique, among them Olympic champions and world record holders Abebe Bikila and Tegla Loroupe, as well as Zola Budd. However, one of the major reasons the barefoot-running trend has taken off was the publication of a research study in the highly respected journal *Nature* by Harvard scientist Daniel E. Lieberman. Dr. Lieberman wrote that that those who run barefoot, or in minimal footwear, tend to avoid "heel-striking," and instead land on the ball of the foot or the middle of the foot. In so doing, these runners use the architecture of the foot and leg and some clever Newtonian physics to avoid hurtful and potentially damaging impacts—equivalent to two to three times body weight—that shod heel-strikers repeatedly experience. To read more about this research study[10], *see the summary on Science Daily.* You can also visit Dr. Lieberman's laboratory website (www.fas.harvard.edu/~skeleton/danlhome.html). Sources: van Gent et al., 2007; *Science Daily.*

If you want to try barefoot running, here are some great tips:

► The landing should feel gentle and relaxed.
► Try to land on the ball of your foot slightly to the outside.
► Try to have your footfall with your foot under your hips or slightly in front. (Striding with your foot too far in front of your body can cause the heel to strike first.)
► Build up very slowly.
► If your feet or calves hurt, stop!

Dr. Lieberman cautioned that a transition to barefoot running should be done gradually. Runners should not increase the distance they run by more than 10% a week, he said, and they should stop and seek medical advice if they experience any pain. "My big worry is that the biggest challenge of barefoot running is that it requires a lot more calf muscle strength and Achilles tendon stretching and people can be prone to Achilles tendonitis if they don't transition gradually and carefully," he said. "It's not for everyone."

related, especially in children with chronic disease. Chronically ill children participate in fewer activities, have lower self-esteem, experience greater anxiety about sports and spend less time exercising As a result of these factors, they are often deconditioned. Sometimes diseases attack muscles either directly or indirectly, often with tragic consequences. My research team has recently shown that lung diseases such as cystic fibrosis actually cause damage to muscle tissue. I described this research in Chapter 1, but now that we have explored muscle physiology it's worth revisiting and evaluating our results in the light of our newly gained understanding of muscle anatomy and physiology.

We were interested in using exercise as a therapy for patients with cystic fibrosis because, although drug and gene therapies have had some benefits, a cure for the disease remains elusive. My colleagues at the Hospital for Sick Children in Toronto have shown that CF patients with higher levels of physical activity have a rate of decline in lung function that is 50% slower than that of patients who don't exercise.[11] These results were independent of disease status. It's not just that sicker kids don't exercise because they're not feeling well and, therefore, they deteriorate faster; but even the "healthier" children with CF who were not active also had great rates of decline in lung function. As part of my post-doctoral training at Sick Kids, I asked children with CF to exercise while inside an MRI machine. A generous donor, Mr. Arnold Irwin, helped us purchase an MRI-compatible cycle ergometer that allowed children to exercise while actually in the MRI. We asked them to do some sprint cycling for 30 seconds to test the high-energy phosphate system and type IIb muscle fibres; 90 seconds of exhausting cycling to test the anaerobic glycolytic system and the type IIa muscle fibres; and, finally, 10 30-second exercise bouts at a moderate level with a few seconds of rest between to test the aerobic system and their type I muscle fibres. We discovered that patients with CF have lower-resting ATP levels, meaning that even when not exercising, the patients have a decreased energy supply. The mechanism for this loss is unknown, but it may be related to the defective protein in CF that's present in the muscle and how it is involved in regulating processes in the muscle cell.

We also discovered that CF patients have higher pH levels at the end of exercise, meaning that they don't accumulate as many hydrogen ions as healthy controls for the same exercise intensity. We think this is because the CF protein defect does not allow for bicarbonate (HCO_3)—an acid buffer in cells and blood—to transfer across the muscle membrane out into the blood as would normally occur in healthy muscle. So bicarbonate levels may be higher in the muscles of patients with CF, and these bicarbonate molecules absorb hydrogen ions (H^+). (Bicarbonate, by the way, is the same substance as the baking soda that people use to absorb refrigerator odours.) This increase in bicarbonate levels in CF patients could be considered a physiological benefit; a higher intracellular bicarbonate concentration could lead to less acid accumulating during high-intensity exercise because bicarbonate "buffers" acid. Therefore, patients with CF may gain more benefit by exercising with short bursts of high-intensity activity; their muscles are predisposed to handle this type of work. Fortunately, the nature of children's play is start–stop. So, despite parents' fears for the health of their child, and perhaps not wanting their child to be outside racing around a playground, this activity is exactly what kids with CF should be doing.

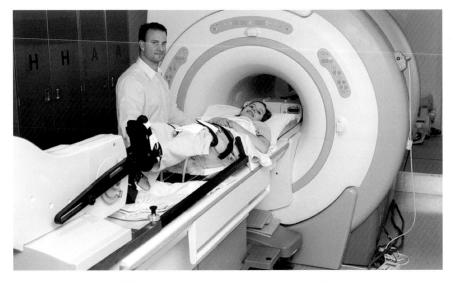

*With recent advances in **MRI** technology, we can now measure chemicals in the body during exercise.*

A group of about 100 diseases cause progressive muscle weakness, defects in muscle proteins and even muscle-cell death. Collectively, this group is often referred to as muscular dystrophies (MD). Often, muscular dystrophies are caused by genetic defects that affect the way muscle proteins are formed and are responsible for the muscle dysfunction. The most common form of MD is Duchenne muscular dystrophy. Researchers have shown that patients with Duchenne's have diminished levels of the protein dystrophin. Dystrophin helps maintain the structure of muscle cells, and when it's not present in sufficient quantities the cell structure and membranes break down. The end result is muscle wasting and weakness. There is currently no cure for MD, although great progress is being made. Exercise can be used as a therapy for patients with MD, as Dr. Paul Vignos from Cleveland's Case Western Reserve University School of Medicine has shown. Dr. Vignos had 24 patients with muscular dystrophy perform strength training using weights for 12 months. He reported that all the patients improved their strength over the first four months of the program, regardless of the type of dystrophy.[12]

But it's not only strength training that has a positive effect on patients with defects of dystrophin. Marie Louise Sveen and her colleagues from the Copenhagen Muscle Research Centre studied the impact of endurance exercise training and found that VO_{2max} increased by 47%, and the maximum work the patients were able to do increased by 80%.[13] Most interestingly, the patients with muscular dystrophy improved 16% more than their matched healthy controls, so the patients with muscle disease were more responsive to training than their healthy counterparts, although this research was done on patients with Becker muscular dystrophy, a less-severe form than Duchenne.

Diabetes also has a negative impact on muscles. With this disease, a lack of the hormone insulin leads to elevated levels of glucose (sugar) in the blood. Insulin works in the body by circulating through the blood and signalling glucose transporters of such target organs as muscles. The glucose transporters pull glucose out of the blood and into the muscle cell, where it is either stored as glycogen for later use or used immediately to help fuel exercise or other metabolic demands. This is why it's necessary to monitor blood-glucose levels and use insulin injections when blood-glucose levels begin to rise. Interestingly, although exercise can't cure diabetes, it can help treat the symptoms and consequences. The benefits of exercise are mostly seen in those at risk of developing type 2 diabetes (the onset of diabetes, often associated with risk factors such as poor diet and low exercise). Exercising muscles are more sensitive to circulating insulin, thus they take up blood glucose more easily and use it more effectively. Further, diabetes is often associated with the buildup of fat molecules in arteries and elsewhere. The buildup of fat is associated with a host of complications. Exercise helps to move and decrease fat stores in the body, and it can even help reverse the onset of type 2 diabetes. As always, if you are looking to start exercising to lessen the effects of any kind of disease, check with your doctor to make sure it is safe to start a program. It's also a great idea to get some advice from a certified fitness professional on establishing a workout program suited to you.

Muscle diseases such as muscular dystrophy affect the protein structure, whereas diabetes affects the ability of the muscle to take in glucose fuel. There can also be genetic defects in the codes for proteins that make up mitochondria. These kinds of diseases are usually referred to as inborn errors of metabolism, or metabolic myopathies. They affect muscle because of the high concentration of mitochondria in muscle tissues, but can also affect the brain, nerves, heart, kidneys and bowel. These mitochondrial diseases usually result in severe weakness and the rapid onset of fatigue.

Muscles can even start to break down, and broken-down muscle components can be found in the blood of patients with metabolic myopathies. The mechanism by which mitochondria do not work properly can, in some cases, be isolated to a part of their oxidative metabolism called the electron transport chain (ETC). The ETC, the final step in the aerobic oxidative pathway, is made up of five proteins located on the membrane (surface) of the mitochondria. These five proteins process hydrogen ions and rebuild adenosine triphospate (ATP), which is then used to fuel muscle contraction. They are made from a specific genetic code; if there's a defect in the code, the proteins are not built with the right structure and a block in the ETC can occur. This block can slow down or stop energy production, depending on the severity of the genetic defect. In 1997, the Nobel Prize for physiology was awarded to the research group that discovered the structure of the ETC. This discovery, in conjunction with other major advances in the fields of muscle physiology, may result in improved treatment for patients with such challenges. Interestingly, exercise therapy does not work well in patients with mitochondrial disease because exercise not only stimulates the production of new mitochondria, but also increases the number and concentration of mitochondria in muscle tissue. As a result, the actual mutant mitochondria may increase and worsen the condition rather than improve it. For now, patients with these types of diseases have to rely on nutritional and pharmacological therapies.

Muscles can also be manipulated to help protect other organs. Dr. Emilie Jean St. Michel, Dr. Andrew Redington and I recently published a study showing a new technique that can improve athletic performance. (This work was based on previous research into a method called preconditioning.) Scientists discovered that by blocking blood flow to muscles for a short time and then allowing it to return (e.g., by inflating a blood pressure cuff above systolic blood pressure to stop blood flow to the arm, and then removing the cuff), it's possible to stimulate the creation and release of an as-yet unidentified molecule that protects the body from subsequent periods of low oxygen supply. Doctors are now using this technique on patients before surgeries on the heart (and other organs) because the circulating molecule appears to protect other organs for hours after reperfusion (blood flow returning to the muscle after circulation was blocked) of the muscle where blood flow was blocked. A study is underway in Denmark, where heart attack patients receive preconditioning in the ambulance on the way to the hospital. Preliminary reports suggest that such preconditioning, applied to the arm of heart attack patients, can reduce the damage to heart muscle even after the heart attack has already started.

Dr. Jean St. Michel, Dr. Reddington and I thought that, since elite-level sport competition is a highly stressful physiological event, perhaps preconditioning athletes before competition would protect their organs and muscles from the metabolic stress of intense exercise. We recently published our results, which showed that preconditioning is related to an improved maximal performance in highly trained swimmers.[15] Swimming seemed like the perfect sport to study, because swimmers can't breathe when they want; they have to limit their breathing to the timing of their stroke. They also spend time underwater around turns, so their blood oxygen levels drop and they can become hypoxic (low-oxygen) during racing. There is also a significant increase in muscle and blood lactic acid levels. So swimming is a physiologically demanding sport that may benefit from the metabolic protection of preconditioning—or so we hypothesized. When we looked at our results, we were amazed to see that preconditioning actually improved athletes' performances in the 100-metre events (these last about 60 seconds) by about 1.5%. This improvement may not seem like much, but for elite athletes it is equivalent to about two years of training. We were able to create this improvement in only one training session. It is critical to note, however, that preconditioning should be attempted only with the assistance of a medical professional. If not done properly, it is very dangerous. *Do not try it at home.*

UNDERSTANDING MUSCLE TRAINING

The great thing about exercise and training is that it doesn't take much to see improvements, and the worse your fitness is to start, the easier it is to make gains. According to the principle of overload, we must exercise at a sufficient intensity in order to stress the body and stimulate adaptation. Well, if you're currently a couch potato, then walking around the block for 15 minutes is pretty stressful physiologically, and your body will improve. If, however, you're an Ironman triathlete, a short walk won't help you much. You'd have to train at or above your second anaerobic threshold to stimulate your body sufficiently. That's the point during exercise when you are working so hard you can hear yourself breathe, or are breathing so hard you can't even speak—according to Dr. Robert Goode from the University of Toronto. But how do we train our muscles to get better? I divide muscle training into three components—muscle endurance, muscle strength and muscle power. Let's work through each one separately.

Muscle-Endurance Training

Muscle endurance can be trained by doing cardiovascular exercises such as running, cycling and swimming. This type of exercise is actually muscle training, but we do thousands of repetitions with very light weights. Think of going for a run. You may take 80 strides per minute (40 steps per leg), where in each stride your leg muscles absorb your body weight and then push off again. This exercise may continue for 30 minutes, and it constitutes a single training set of 1200 repetitions. It is extreme muscle endurance training and is highly effective at improving your cardiovascular system and your type I aerobic oxidative muscle fibres. We can do similar things in the gym to accomplish related physiological goals. Muscle-endurance training requires lifting light weights for repetitions in the 20–30 range with minimal rest. So a typical set of exercises for muscle endurance may look like the following:

SETS	REPETITIONS	REST	WEIGHT
3	20	30 seconds	Enough to make your muscles burn at reps 18–20

Note: A rep is the number of times you repeat an action (e.g., 8 push-ups), and a set is the number of times you do your 8 reps. As an example, you could do 3 sets each of 8 reps. (In total, you would have 24 push-ups.)

We also recommend a consistent tempo for muscle-endurance training—for example, we'd ask the person doing the repetitions to lower the weight in 1 second, then hold for 1 second, then lift the weight in 1 second. This is written as "Tempo 1:1:1."

Another way to endurance train in the gym is to do something called circuit training. You do a number of exercises that work different muscle groups, one set at a time, one after the other. For example, you could start with an exercise that works the chest and arm muscles; move to lunges, which work your legs; then move back to the upper body by doing some push-ups. This plan creates a longer period of constant exercise but allows the muscles in your legs to rest while you work your arms, and vice versa.

Muscle-Strength Training

To increase muscle strength, you have to perform some pretty tough work in the gym using specific equipment. The objective of strength training is to create micro-tears in the muscle fibres so that the body is stimulated to make the muscles stronger to better withstand the stress in the future. These micro-tears, and the molecules that are produced during strength training, stimulate the production of new myosin and actin protein chains—and the muscles grow in size (hypertrophy).

Effective training for increased strength involves moving an object with mass (weight) through a distance by exerting a force on it. In physics, this process is called work. The weight must be heavy enough to cause some micro-damage in the muscle fibres, so, near the end of the set, lift enough weight to make your muscles burn. The repetition range shown to stimulate hypertrophy most effectively is between eight and 12 repetitions. The other key factor in strength training is to take advantage of a type of muscle contraction called eccentric contraction. Eccentric contractions are used to control a weight as the muscle lengthens. For example, if you do a bench press, the muscles in your triceps and the muscles in your chest *lengthen* as you *lower* the weights. They are contracting to control the descent, but they are lengthening at the same time. This contraction, which puts lots of stress on the myofibrils and the contractile apparatus of the muscle, is a powerful stimulus for hypertrophy.

Eccentric muscle contractions will also make you *very* sore, which in this case is a good thing. Just don't lift heavier weights until your muscles are completely recovered and you no longer feel sore. The opposite kind of muscle contraction is called a concentric contraction. It occurs when the muscles shorten. The triceps and pectoral muscles exert a concentric contraction when we lift a weight. A typical training set for strength development will look like this:

SETS	REPETITIONS	REST	WEIGHT
3–6	8–12	90–120 seconds	Enough to make your muscles burn at reps 8–12

Tempos for strength sets can be slow, pause then fast. This would mean taking three seconds to lower the weight and, after a short pause, contracting quickly to lift it. This tempo maximizes the eccentric contraction and also helps build some power in the concentric contraction phase. We'll talk about power in the next section. The tempo for strength workouts is 3 down : 1 hold : 1 up.

Strength training is also great for people looking to improve their body composition and lose fat. Muscles are the tissue in the body that burn fat most easily, so if we can increase our muscle mass, we will have more metabolically active tissue that can burn fat as fuel, even at rest. This component of weight management is the one that most people take the least advantage of, because they're afraid that, by lifting weights, they're going to get big and bulky. Although this may happen in extreme cases like bodybuilding, most people who lift weights for strength development simply improve their body composition (lose fat and gain muscle), feel better and slow the aging process—and this training can be accomplished without getting big, bulky muscles. One thing to remember when monitoring your progress is that muscle weighs more than fat. So when you do strength training, you may gain some weight, even if you are losing fat. However, overall you're improving body composition and health, so this is one type of weight gain that's okay.

GREG'S HIGH-PERFORMANCE TIPS
REDUCING BMI IN KIDS

Recent research by Dr. Catherine Birken at the Hospital for Sick Children in Toronto found that interventions focused only on reducing screen time (computer, TV, etc.) had no effect on reducing body mass index (BMI) in children. Dr. Birken suggests that, to improve body composition in people with obesity, approaches should include healthy nutrition, increased physical activity *and* reduced sedentary activity such as sitting in front of a screen.[16]

Muscle-Power Training

One aspect of muscle training that is often neglected in the strength-endurance dichotomy of training is power—the ability to generate force rapidly. It's a problem I've encountered in my work with the Canadian national golf team. Usually, athletes focus on getting stronger and building bulk, but then they slow down and can't move quickly. In the case of golf, they can't hit the ball as far.

Power is the ability to move an object quickly. Unlike the strength training discussed earlier, there's a time component where speed is involved. Think of jumping, throwing or even sprinting. These activities depend on muscle power, which is a critical factor in many sports. So training for increased muscle power means we have to think of muscle training in a completely different way—really light weights are the key! You just have to move them fast. Medicine balls are used for this type of training because you can throw them around or back and forth to a partner. Boxing training is gaining popularity. In this case, you are asked to box—or move your hands and arms as quickly as possible—and the only weight you have is the gloves. This type of exercise provides some of the most exhausting training out there—but it's also really, really fun! Here is how exercises can be designed to do power training:

SETS	REPETITIONS	REST	WEIGHT
3–6	4–6	90–120 seconds	Light enough to be able to move the weight quickly, but still results in muscle strain on reps 4–6.

Specific weight-training sessions to develop power incorporate light loads (similar to muscular endurance training), but the weights must be lifted at explosive velocities. Therefore, jumping and medicine ball exercises can also used.

Because power workouts involve speed and explosiveness, getting professional guidance is a key to success and avoiding injury—always check with a certified strength coach or fitness professional before trying these exercises. Moving at speed increases your risk of injury, so preparing for this type of training often takes months or even years. But it's a good goal to have because, as I mentioned, it's completely different and lots of fun. I've developed a Power Pyramid Model that can be used to guide the development of an athlete, or anyone else who is interested in muscle training. It is shown in the figure that follows.

In this model, we start with training at the base of the pyramid, learning movements and building base muscle endurance. Strengthening the core muscles is also critical at the base stage, because strong abdominal, hip and back muscles help stabilize the body for the more complicated and faster movements used later in the muscle development pathway. I recommend that, once an acceptable level of base muscle endurance training and core stability has been developed, people move into building muscle strength. This training helps you create new muscle tissue and develop enough maximal strength so you're capable of moving at higher speeds and forces without injury. It also stimulates the tendons that connect muscles to the bones to get stronger. At the top of the pyramid is the power development area, where individuals can work on agility, speed and explosiveness. As for athletes, each stage of the pyramid can take about 10 to 12 weeks within the context a single season. But we can also look at training in terms of overall athletic development, where each stage can take up to a few years to perfect. Under the supervision of a fitness professional, non-athlete readers of this book can use the power pyramid to guide their training program design, with each of the four stages taking anywhere from 6 to 12 weeks, depending on one's fitness level.

Power Pyramid Model

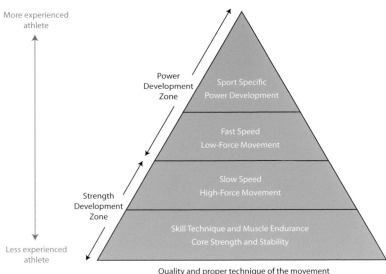

More experienced athlete

Power Development Zone

Sport Specific Power Development

Fast Speed Low-Force Movement

Strength Development Zone

Slow Speed High-Force Movement

Skill Technique and Muscle Endurance Core Strength and Stability

Less experienced athlete

Quality and proper technique of the movement is of **highest** importance at all levels of the pyramid

HOW TO CHALLENGE YOUR CORE MUSCLES DURING YOUR WORKOUT

The key to challenging your core muscles, and therefore stimulating them to become stronger and more effective at stabilizing your body during movements, is to create "unbalanced" training situations. For example, the traditional bench press can be used to work the pectorals and triceps when done on a bench with a bar. But if you do this exercise on a stability ball using dumbbells, then the exercise suddenly expands to include the pectoral muscles, the triceps, the rotator cuff muscles, the glutes and all the abdominal muscles.

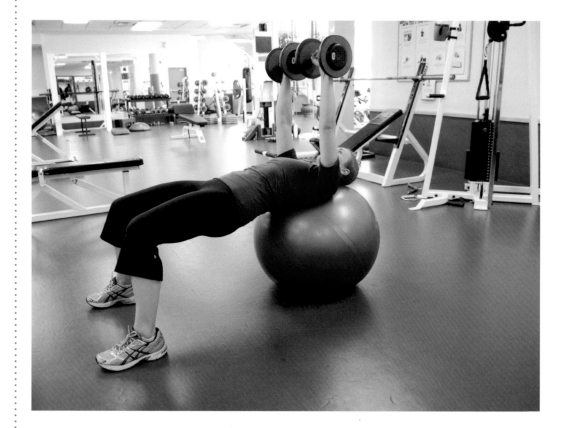

Instructions. Grab two dumbbells, one for each hand, and sit on a stability ball. Stabilizing the dumbbells on your chest, slowly walk yourself out on the ball until it is directly under your mid-back. From here, raise both dumbbells directly up in front of your chest. Now, try to perform a chest press with both arms—lowering the dumbbells to your chest and returning them to the extended position. Make sure you stabilize your core as you perform the chest press. For an added challenge to the core muscles, you can try doing this exercise one arm at a time, now lowering one dumbbell while keeping the other in the raised position. Always do this exercise with a partner to spot you, because it's easy to lose your balance. Also, begin this exercise using very light weights, and progress slowly toward more challenging weights.

Another way to increase the complexity of your exercises and increase the contribution of core muscles to the execution of the movement is by modifying the way push-ups are done. Once again, the principle is to create an unbalanced situation, where more muscles have to be engaged for the exercise to be completed successfully.

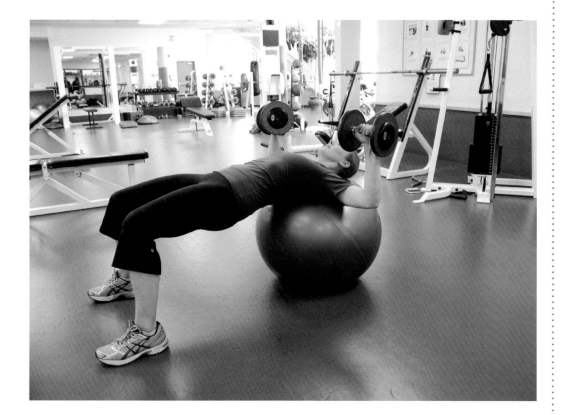

Here is a normal push-up:

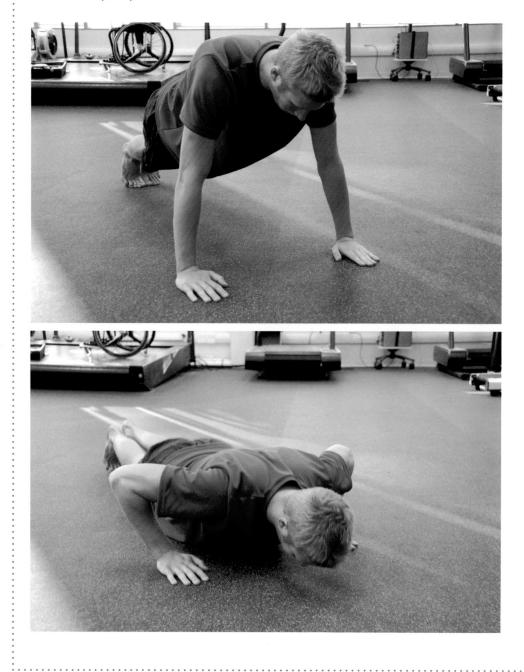

By placing a medicine ball (6 kilograms in this case) under one arm during the movement, the body becomes slightly unbalanced and complementary muscles are engaged.

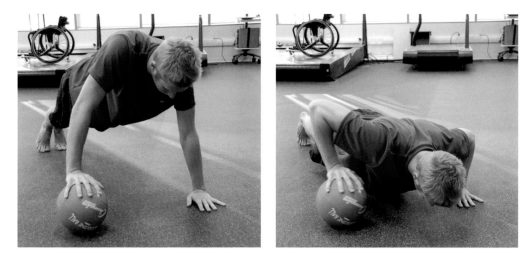

In this further modification, the medicine ball is placed under both hands (be careful!). This exercise is highly challenging, but it's an excellent one for shoulder stability strength and core muscle activation.

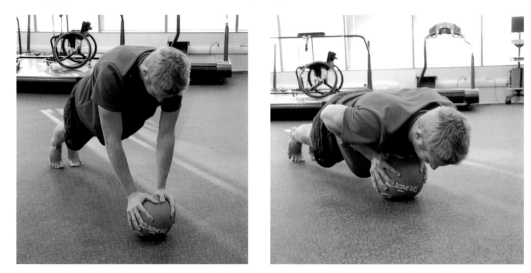

The possibilities for changing traditional exercises to make them more challenging are endless. Talk to a professional fitness trainer or strength-training coach to make sure that you learn how to do the exercises properly and safely.

The Difference between Muscle Endurance, Strength and Power Training

Muscle-resistance training is challenging but lots of fun, and it provides you with some powerful results. There are significant differences between the three types of training, and that works out well. Although you may be in the gym lifting weights, you can do very different workouts with very different effects. Athletes use these different modes of training to build up capacity in various physical areas, and you can do the same if you execute the movements properly. Here are some examples of the same exercise being performed very differently. Let's start with a foundational exercise that's part of many people's training programs—the squat.

The squat is a great exercise because it is so fundamental—we squat all the time. It also activates many muscle groups in the body, so it's an efficient exercise in that it develops muscle capacities in many areas of the body simultaneously. It is also one of the easiest exercises for injuring yourself, so make sure to first get professional coaching on how to do it. If you accept this challenge, here's how to perform the squat to train muscle endurance, strength and power.

First, if you use light weights and perform more than 15 repetitions, this exercise can be highly effective in increasing the endurance capacities of the body's muscles. Here's elite sport trainer Adrian Li demonstrating a squat with minimal weight.

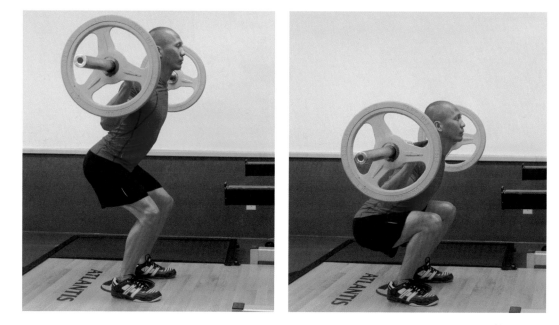

To change this exercise to one where hypertrophy is stimulated and strength is increased, the repetitions can be decreased to between 8 and 12, and the weight increased. Here Adrian has added some weights to the bar (you can see the red and yellow weights now, and the strain on his face as he is lifting).

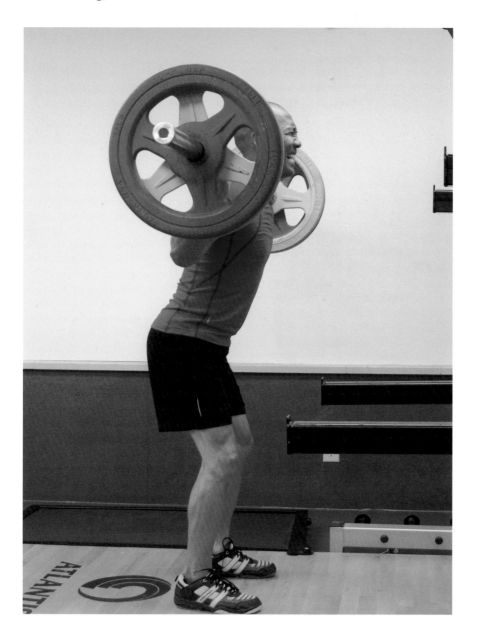

Finally, to create a movement where you are training explosive power, speed is the key. So the repetitions can be decreased to between 4 and 6, and the weight can be decreased as well to ensure that the movement is happening as quickly as possible. Here Adrian is using a very light weight on the bar. He's contracted his muscles so powerfully that he is in fact doing a jump.

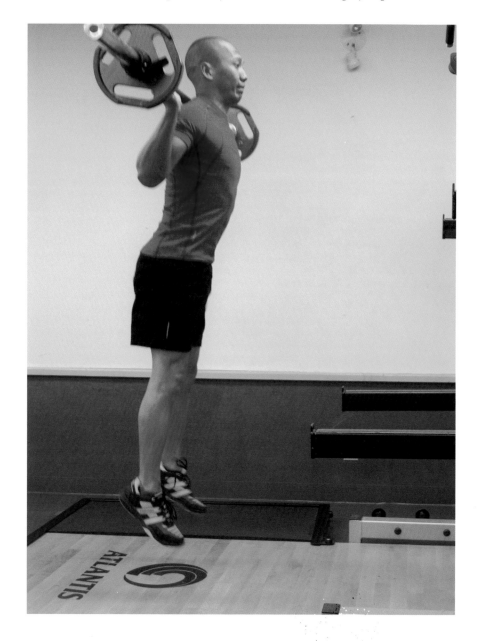

The same modifications can be made to other exercises. In this case, for endurance training, chin-ups can be done with no weight. (You can even do this exercise on an assisted machine, which most gyms have, or use some surgical tubing to get a lift—chin-ups are hard.)

With some practice and initial training, you can add weights and increase the resistance to train for strength.

And with lots of training and motivation, you can do a few reps at very high energy outputs to train for power. In this case, Adrian has actually pulled himself up so fast that he can let go of the bar for a moment, before catching and lowering himself to the ground.

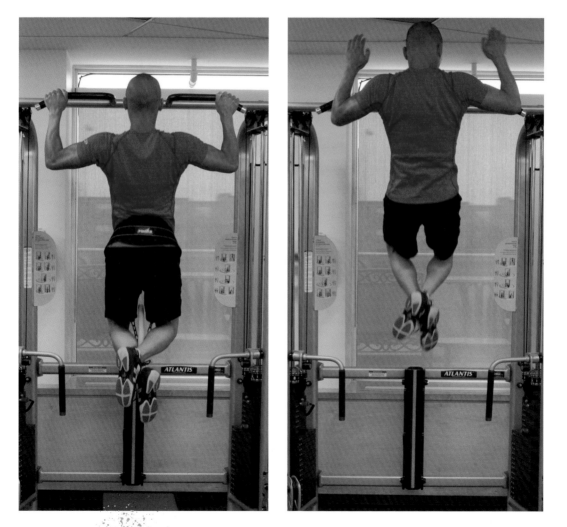

Even the most basic exercises can be modified this way. You can do unloaded push-ups (you can even do these from your knees, if necessary). Try to keep the repetitions high to train muscle endurance.

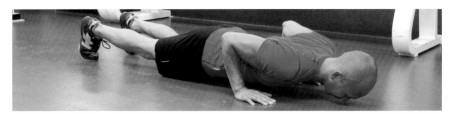

More resistance can be added by placing a weight on the back. As I mentioned, make sure you do this under the supervision of a professional strength coach. Also use light weights to start, and have someone spot you to make sure the weight stays in a safe position. Keep your core activated constantly to prevent injuries to your lower back.

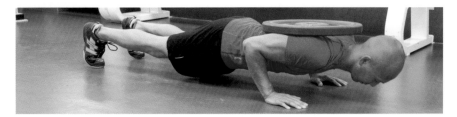

Power training with push-ups can be quite fun. Simply try to push upward as quickly as possible. In this case, Adrian has propelled himself off the ground and is clapping his hands. Keep the repetitions low so that muscle speed is the focus.

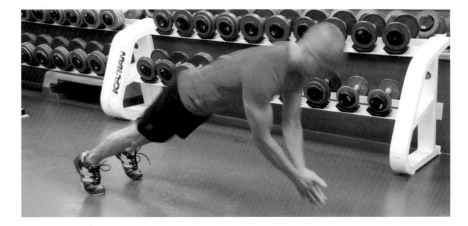

You can use this knowledge to develop challenging, effective and enjoyable muscle-training programs. Have fun and feel free to comment or ask questions on Facebook (www.facebook.com/gregwellsphd) or Twitter @drgregwells.

SUMMARY OF MUSCLE-TRAINING WORKOUT DESIGN

MUSCULAR ENDURANCE—the ability of a muscle (or muscle group) to continually exert force against resistance

Sets:	3–5
Repetitions:	15–30
Tempo:	Eccentric 1 : Pause 1 : Concentric 1
Rest:	30–90 seconds between each set
Frequency:	3–4 times per week, with a minimum of 24 hours' recovery

MUSCLE STRENGTH AND HYPERTROPHY—the increase in muscle cell size and the ability of a muscle (or muscle group) to maximally exert force against resistance

Sets:	3–6
Repetitions:	8–12
Tempo:	Eccentric 3 : Pause 1 : Concentric 1
Rest:	90 seconds to 3 minutes between each set
Frequency:	2–3 times per week, with a minimum of 48 hours' recovery

MUSCLE POWER—the amount of work done per unit of time

Sets:	1–5
Repetitions:	4–6
Tempo:	Eccentric 1–2 : Pause 1 : Concentric <1
Rest:	3+ minutes between sets; can do light cardio between sets
Frequency:	1–2 times per week, with a minimum of 72 hours' recovery

Remember, the recommended post-workout recovery fuel after strength training is a mixture of carbohydrates and proteins with a ratio of 2:1 carbs to proteins. I also suggest omega-3s after a power workout to help the nervous system recover.

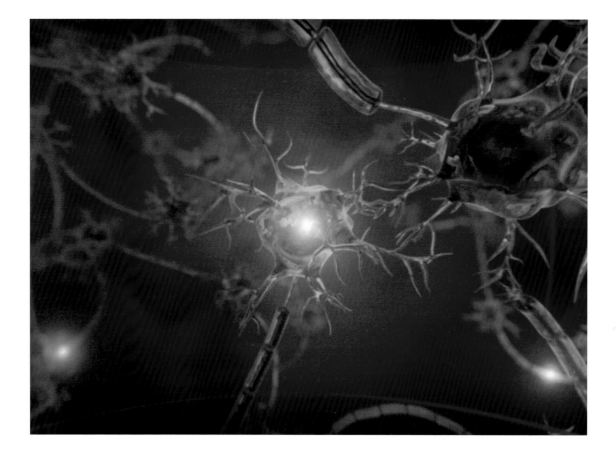

ENERGIZING YOUR BRAIN

THE NERVOUS SYSTEM

3

Many children grow up participating in sports, and I was lucky to be one of the kids whose parents gave them the opportunity to pursue their dreams. When I was 15, I was a member of Canada's national youth swimming team and training as hard as I could to pursue my dream of making the Olympics. My swim team went to a training camp in Florida, and on the second day a group of us decided to go for a swim in the ocean before heading to a meet in the afternoon. We started body surfing and playing in the waves, because we were super comfortable in the water and, at 15, thought we were invincible. That morning I learned I was not invincible when a big wave picked me up and dropped me on my head. I broke several vertebrae and tore ligaments in my neck. Fortunately, my neck muscles went into spasm and protected my shattered spine until I got to the hospital, where I was admitted. That moment led to three months of traction, neurosurgery and rehabilitation. Thanks to my parents, friends, school and teammates, I was able to work hard and get back to race in the Olympic trials 16 months after the injury.

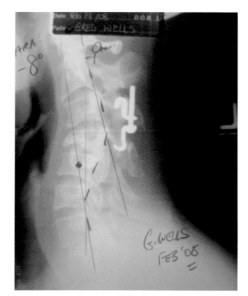

That process started my lifelong interest in the nervous system and how it works when it's healthy and also when it's broken.

BREAKTHROUGH IN SPINAL CORD REPAIR RESEARCH

In research published in the highly regarded journal *Nature,* Dr. Katherine Zukor and Dr. Zhigang He from the Kirby Program in Neuroscience, Children's Hospital Boston, explain how they have successfully repaired damaged spinal cords in mice, restoring the animals' ability to breathe after spinal cord injury. The scientists used new techniques that promote the neurons' ability to repair themselves (called plasticity) and regenerate connections that have been broken. This research offers hope to people who have suffered spinal cord injuries above the level of the fourth cervical vertebra and require the assistance of a ventilator to breathe.[17]

The brain is so complicated that we will likely never uncover all its mysteries. The human brain has 100 billion neurons, with 100 trillion connections between them. These neurons are responsible for everything from our senses to our thoughts and memories. Because our thoughts, emotions, memories and movements are created, organized and controlled by these nerves and synaptic connections, the potential of the human brain appears to be unlimited. The central nervous system, which consists of the brain and the spinal cord, is the control system for the entire body. The cerebellum, a bundle of nerves on the back of the brain that looks a bit like a cauliflower, is where movements are coordinated. Our spinal cord carries electrical signals down to our bodies, where links to the peripheral nervous system then take the information from our brains out to the target organs, including the muscles.

The peripheral nervous system (PNS) is the system of nerves that connects the spinal cord to all the organs (including the muscles) and glands in the human body. It carries information and messages from the spinal cord to the target organs. The PNS also carries messages from sensory receptors in organs and structures back to the spinal cord and, thereby, to the brain.

The peripheral nervous system can be subdivided into two primary subsystems—the somatic and autonomic components. Think of the somatic system as the nerves that are under your voluntary control and connected to your skeletal muscles. The autonomic system, which is not usually under conscious control, is connected to internal organs and blood vessels. This system is further subdivided into the sympathetic nervous system, which increases activation of the target tissue or organ, and the parasympathetic system, which acts to calm down the tissues or organs. For example, when the sympathetic system is active, the smooth muscles in your eyes cause

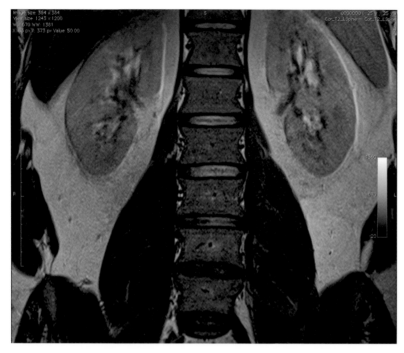

An **MRI** of the lower back, showing the spinal cord, the vertebrae, the disks and the kidneys.

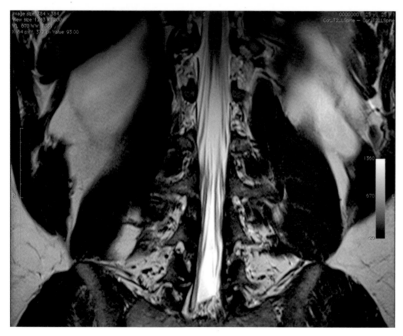

This **MRI** shows the nerves in the spinal cord.

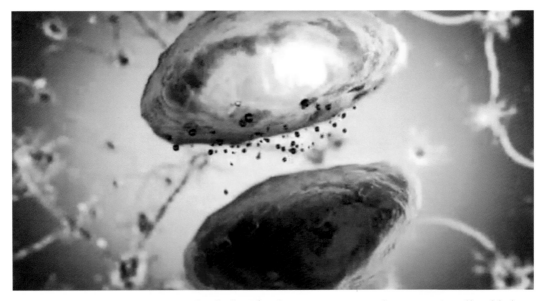

This image shows how nerves communicate with each other. When the synapse receives a signal, neurotransmitters (the red dots) are released, carrying the signal from the end of one nerve to the end of the other.

your irises to dilate (grow bigger); conversely, the parasympathetic system will act to relax those smooth muscles and the irises will contract. The organization of the nervous system is complicated, but will make a lot of sense if you look at it as an organization chart for a business.

Electrical signals are carried from the brain through the central nervous system and peripheral nervous systems out to the muscle. When the electrical signals arrive at the muscle, they trigger the release of chemical messengers from the nerve endings, called neurotransmitters. There are three main types of neurotransmitters in the central nervous system: amino acids (e.g., glutamate and gamma-Aminobutyric acid [GABA]); peptides (including vasopressin and somatostatin, among others); and monoamines (such as norepinephrine, dopamine, serotonin and acetylcholine). GABA, a neurotransmitter that is widely distributed throughout the brain cortex, is involved in motor control, vision and anxiety. Glutamate is a major neurotransmitter in the brain and is associated with learning and memory. Acetylcholine (ACh) activates the motor neurons that control skeletal muscles. Dopamine (DA), another neurotransmitter found primarily in the brain, is related to the control of voluntary movement and pleasurable emotions. Serotonin (5-HT) is involved in the regulation of sleep, wakefulness, appetite, pain, mood and aggression. Norepinephrine is a neurotransmitter that is important for attentiveness, emotions, sleeping, dreaming and learning. It also acts as a hormone since it can be released into the blood, where it causes the blood vessels to contract and the heart rate to increase. Only acetylcholine and norepinephrine are found in the peripheral nervous system. If the nerve connection happens to be with a muscle, then the neurotransmitter signal causes a series of events that result in the muscle contracting. As we'll see in a moment, this is what occurred when Usain Bolt broke the world record in the 100-metre dash at the 2008 Olympics.

When we reach for a glass of water, we hardly think about it. But even this simple movement results in a flurry of electrical and chemical activity in the brain, spinal cord and peripheral nervous system. Let's look at Usain Bolt's world record 9.58-second 100-metre dash. Exploring "the start" is fascinating when we consider the lighting storm of electrical activity involved. There are three steps to the start: the "On Your Mark," "Get Set" and "Go" steps. These are followed by two critical stages of the race: the acceleration phase and the speed maintenance phase. Let's take a look at each of these steps.

GREG'S HIGH-PERFORMANCE TIPS

NERVES

Nerves that carry signals to the muscles to move are called motor neurons, and nerves that carry information back to the spinal cord are called sensory neurons. For example, nerve signals will travel from the spinal cord, through motor nerves, to muscles—where the nerve signals will result in the initiation of a muscle contraction. This muscle contraction will cause joints to move, and the peripheral nerves that sense movement in muscle and joints (these nerves are called proprioceptors—more on them later) will send information back to the spinal cord through sensory nerves, informing the brain about what is happening to the body.

ON YOUR MARK!

When Usain Bolt approached the blocks and placed himself in the position to start the race, he was still physically relaxed, but his brain was actively preparing to run. The parietal and frontal lobes of the brain were preparing the appropriate physical activities and making decisions about the motor activities about to happen. The prefrontal cortex was making plans about how to execute the start and to run a world-record race. The frontal cortex was receiving information from axons (which are connected to the parietal lobe) regarding the spatial orientation of all the muscles, limbs and joints in the body. The activation of the motor areas of the brain occurred because of the nerve impulses coming through sensory nerves from the ears and eyes, which provide information about the environment. The crowd noises stimulated the auditory

TRAINING YOUR MOTOR PATTERNS IS THE KEY TO GREAT TECHNIQUE

Motor patterns are important because they're a sequence of events that the nervous system uses to create movements. With practice, these patterns become more efficient and ingrained, which means that we can rely on them to execute movements. The downside is that if we learn or practise a movement with poor technique, improper motor patterns are created and reinforced. So if you're learning a new skill or practising an old one, maintain great technique as often as possible.

nerves, and the sights of the stadium activated the visual nerves and related areas of the brain. This information was synthesized to determine the best reactions to plan and execute. Further, at this point the sympathetic nervous system—which acts to dilate blood vessels, increase heart rate and breathing, and pump glucose into the bloodstream—was being activated.

GET SET!

As soon as the starter said "Set," the premotor areas of the brain, located in the back of the frontal lobe, built the exact strategies for the movement in preparation for the upcoming execution of the start. The brain made calculations about the coordinates of the starting blocks, the track and the finish line, and worked with the cerebellum to plan and calibrate the required movements. The cerebellum is the air-traffic controller for signals related to movements that pass from the back of the frontal lobes (areas where motor function and movements are controlled) to and from the spinal cord. There are so many neurons in the cerebellum that, although it makes up only 10% of the brain's total volume, it accounts for more than 50% of its neurons. The cerebellum also acts as a learning centre for movement patterns. As it receives (from the proprioceptors) input on the joints and muscles of the limbs, it constantly compares the actual movements made by the body with the planned movements that were called for by the brain before the initiation of the movement. So the movement patterns that we execute—such as throwing a baseball or, in this case, running—get calibrated over time and become increasingly refined.

For the beautiful movements of sports to happen, the brain, nerve pathways and muscles must all work in a coordinated and sequenced manner. The integrated signals from the brain through to the muscle contraction that create movement are called a motor pattern. Well-developed motor patterns that have been refined over years of practice are why great athletes make sports look so easy. Each movement—and there are no extra ones—is perfectly programmed and refined. Think of a world-class diver repeating the same exacting, fluid movements thousands of times throughout a career

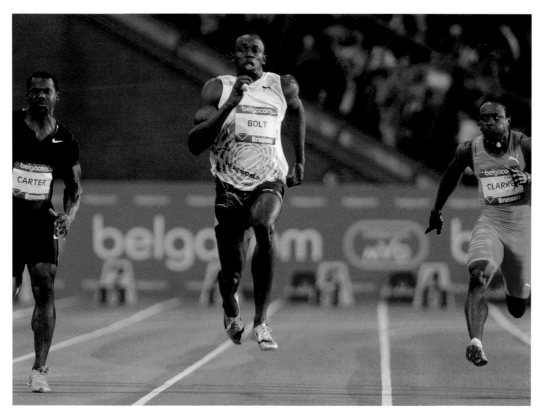

Usain Bolt, the world's fastest man, looks like he's flying down the track. During the 10-second event he's in contact with the ground for less than 4 seconds. Sprinters have some of the most highly developed nervous systems of all athletes.

in order to compete at the highest level. The performance appears effortless, but only because years of training have refined the motor patterns that are stored in the brain and coordinated in the cerebellum so that movements are fluid and efficient. The cerebellum learns how to calibrate the signals that it commands to the muscles to control the duration and strength of the stimulus and, thus, the precision of the movement. As Usain Bolt holds his start position in the blocks, motor patterns that have been programmed through thousands of repetitions over years of practice and training are about to be activated.

GO!

As soon as the starter's gun goes off, a flurry of activity begins. Motor commands from the motor cortex at the back of the frontal lobe are considered by the cerebellum. The final movement commands are then sent

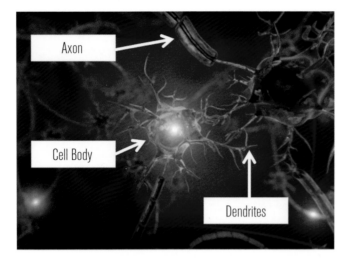

Axon

Cell Body

Dendrites

The parts of a nerve.

down the spinal cord and from there to the peripheral nervous system and the motor neurons.

The fundamental component of the brain and the nervous system is the neuron. This is a specialized cell that consists of three main components—the dendrites, the cell body and the axon. The dendrites are branches of the neuron that connect to other neurons and receive signals, which they carry back to the cell body. The cell body, which is the main part of the neuron, contains the nucleus, DNA and mitochondria, among other components. The axon carries electrical signals from the cell body to other neurons or to target organs such as muscle cells. Axons vary in size, from microscopic lengths in the brain to nearly two metres long if they run all the way to the legs.

Although signals can pass through their own dendrites and axons at extremely high speeds (from 3 to 300 kilometres per hour), communication between neurons (or target organs) happens chemically at a much slower pace. When the electrical signal arrives at the junction between neurons or between the neuron and the muscle (called a nerve terminal), it triggers a series of events that result in the release of neurotransmitters into the space between the originating nerve and the target organ. This space is called a synapse.

When signals pass across the synapse, the signal from the originating nerve can (1) trigger a new nerve impulse if it is a neuron-to-neuron connection; (2) trigger a muscle contraction if it is a nerve-to-muscle connection; or (3) trigger the release of a hormone from an endocrine gland if it is a nerve-to–endocrine gland connection. Neurotransmitters carry the signal between the originating nerve and the adjacent nerve or target organ.

The actual contraction of the muscle fibres is initiated by the release of the neurotransmitter acetylcholine into the synaptic gap in the neuromuscular junction. The acetylcholine travels across the synapse and binds to receptors on the muscle fibre. This action triggers channels in the membranes of the muscle to release calcium, which diffuses into the myofibrils and initiates the binding of actin and myosin filaments—and,

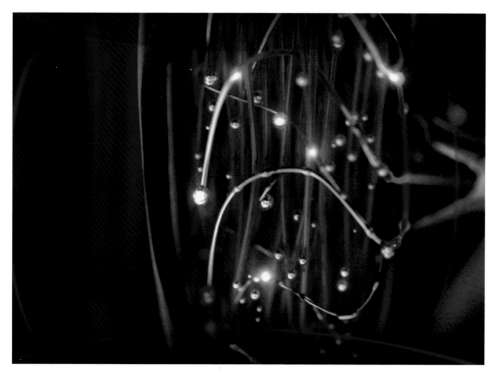

*An artist's rendition of a golgi tendon organ (**GTO**), a special nerve that senses the development of force inside tendons. **GTO**s initiate a reflex that automatically bypasses the brain and causes muscles to contract, protecting the muscles and tendons from tearing.*

thereby, muscle contraction. At that point, Usain Bolt is off and running to a world record.

THE ACCELERATION PHASE

A special type of movement takes advantage of the nervous system to supercharge muscles. Each time that Usain Bolt's foot struck the ground during the acceleration phase of his 100-metre dash, he took advantage of this reaction, called plyometrics. You've probably experienced the plyometric reaction in your doctor's office during your annual physical exam. Remember when your doctor takes out his little mallet and taps your patellar tendon right below the knee? Your quadriceps muscle and the tendons that connect the muscle to bone stretch very quickly, thanks to this motion. The sudden lengthening of your muscle sets off what is called the stretch reflex. That reflex is modulated by two special nerve fibres—muscle spindles and golgi tendon organs (GTO).

Muscle spindles are sensory receptors that wrap around muscle fibres and detect changes in the length of the muscle. So if you *slowly* move your muscle through a range of motion, the muscle spindles will not sense any danger and will remain "silent." If, however, the muscle tendon complex lengthens quickly, then the muscle spindles fire signals back to the central nervous system. These signals activate alpha motoneurons, leading back to the muscle that's being lengthened. Similarly, golgi tendon organs, which are located in the area where the tendons link to the muscle, are sensitive to the force that's developed. Both muscle spindles and golgi tendon organs serve as protection mechanisms that likely evolved to prevent muscles and tendons from being torn or damaged. When the signal reaches the spinal cord, immediate signals are sent back to the muscle along the neurons that are connected to muscles—the process takes less than 0.02 seconds. The muscle responds by contracting, and that's why you see your leg kick up right after your doctor hits your patellar tendon with that little mallet. The really cool aspect of this response is that it's one of the few movements happening in the human body that totally bypasses the brain. Sending the signal back to the brain would take too long to effectively protect the muscle.

Each time Usain Bolt's toes and the ball of his foot hit the ground, his Achilles tendon and calf muscle fibres were placed on stretch very quickly. This position would have stretched the elastic components of the muscle tissue (connective tissue and fascia, for example). But it may also have quickly stretched the muscle fibres and activated the plyometric reflex, thereby increasing the force of the muscle contraction that then propelled him down the track.

The plyometric reaction can be seen in many sports. Basketball players demonstrate it when they explode off the ground before dunking a ball. Among track and field athletes, it appears the moment before takeoff on high jump. It's seen in mogul skiing and in the explosive movements of gymnastics. In these critical moments, muscles are loaded very quickly during an eccentric contraction (when the muscle is contracting and lengthening at the same time); then, using the plyometric contract in addition to powerful motor signals from the brain, they contract concentrically very quickly to generate the power that the athletes need to execute their moves.

Plyometric training, which involves putting a muscle on stretch before actively contracting it, originated in the Eastern bloc countries in the 1970s. Although the sports scientists in East Germany and the Soviet

Union used doping methods that were not only unethical but also seriously damaged the health of their athletes, some of the advances these researchers made were ethical and cutting edge, and they heightened our knowledge of how the human body can be trained for improved athletic performance. Because the forces that are created during plyometrics are so great, caution must be taken when attempting this type of exercise. If you're interested in trying this form of training, make sure you consult a qualified therapist, coach or trainer to be certain you are strong enough to do the movements safely and learn the proper technique.

The benefits of plyometric training are significant. Among volleyball players, figure skaters and gymnasts, it has been clearly shown to increase vertical jump height more than

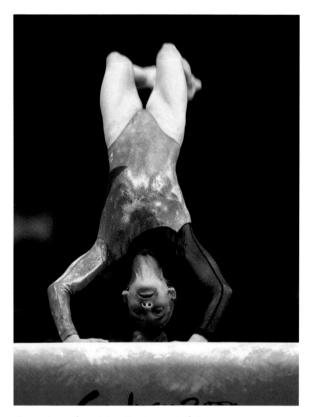

Gymnasts use plyometric action to execute their moves.

strength training alone. Because the forces that pass through the body are great, plyometric training has also been shown to stimulate bone density, so it's particularly good not only for female athletes, but also for women in general who want to build up their bone health. And, perhaps most importantly, it's a lot of fun and very different from more traditional types of training.

MAINTENANCE OF MAXIMUM-VELOCITY PHASE—FIGHTING FATIGUE FOR THE WIN

The critical phase of the 100-metre dash is the maintenance of speed phase when athletes fight metabolic and neural fatigue. Most if not all athletes actually decelerate during the 100-metre dash, even though it lasts only 9.58+ seconds and the athlete who wins is usually the one who decelerates the least. Inside the body, it comes down to the athlete with the best resistance to fatigue—and the nervous system, just like muscle, is subject to fatigue factors. During exercise the brain sends signals to the muscles,

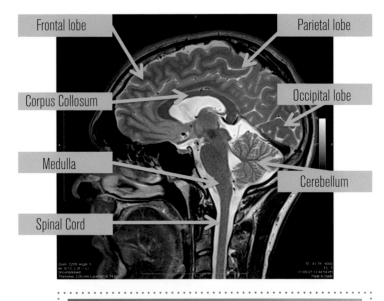

Frontal lobe

Parietal lobe

Corpus Collosum

Occipital lobe

Medulla

Cerebellum

Spinal Cord

directing them to contract and helping us to perform. In addition to those nerves which take information to the muscles that initiate and control movement, there are many nerves that collect information about the state of the muscles, blood vessels and other structures and relay that information back to the brain. This feed-forward and feedback system serves to regulate and control exercise intensity. Some scientists believe that the communication between the brain and the body is what ultimately limits exercise performance. They have termed this process the central fatigue hypothesis. In this case, the word "central" refers to the brain as the master controller for exercise intensity in the body.

The brain is the most complicated organ in the human body. Although we are only beginning to understand how the brain works, scientists have established the main roles of its different areas. (Note, however, that new research shows that the brain's roles can change. Check out "The Brain That Changes Itself" by Dr. Norman Doige.[18]) The frontal lobes of the brain are where emotions, personality, problem-solving, memory, language, judgment, and social and sexual behaviours are controlled. The parietal lobe is involved with sensations, perception and integration of information from the visual system. The two parts of the parietal lobe act to integrate sensory information to form a single perception and cognition of the world around us—to create "spatial awareness" so that we can coordinate our movements within our physical environment. The temporal lobe is also involved with integrating auditory and visual sensory information as well as memory and language. The cerebellum acts to coordinate movements, while the medulla maintains vital body functions, such as breathing and heart rate.

THE BRAIN AND PSYCHOLOGICAL STRESS

In October 2010, the world watched as thirty-three miners emerged from under the Atacama Desert in Chile after having been trapped underground for four months. The miners became stuck when a tunnel collapsed, and they had to wait until an escape route could be drilled down to the space in which they were waiting. They survived in a small area (700 metres) the size of a living room, where conditions were highly challenging. There was limited space to exercise, and it was 32°C in the area where they were trapped. Furthermore, since there are no light/dark cues below the surface, their circadian rhythms became disrupted.

The psychological stress that the miners faced in the first days after being trapped must have been severe—a factor that would have activated their sympathetic nervous systems. This system is designed to prepare for immediate activity (fight or flight) in response to a perceived threat or stress. The parasympathetic system implements rest and recovery, helping the internal organ systems to relax. You can see the opposite effects of these two systems in the figure on page 83.

You can easily understand the sympathetic and parasympathetic systems just by thinking about what happens to you if you're stressed or nervous. When you're stressed, all the physical reactions on the right side of the figure happen within seconds, but if you take some time to relax and calm down, then the parasympathetic system becomes dominant and the organ systems relax, as in the left side of the figure.

The activation of the sympathetic nervous system causes the release of fight or flight hormones from the adrenal glands, which sit right above the kidneys. Adrenaline and norepinephrine impair digestion, ready the body for activity and slow down some aspects of the immune system. Noradrenaline has been shown to strengthen neuron connections in the brain that create memories related to stressful, emotional or traumatic events—the opposite responses of those needed to keep the miners alive and healthy.

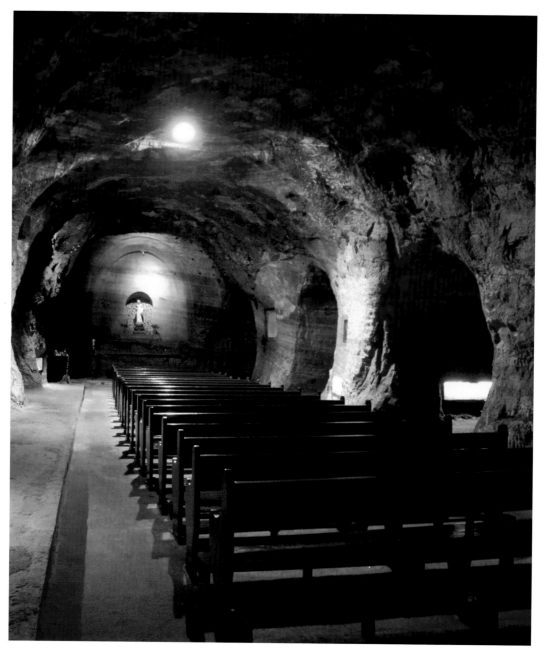

Miners are acutely aware of the dangers of their jobs. The day the miners emerged from below the surface, I was at a conference in Bogotá, Colombia. The organizers took me to visit a local salt mine. All the way down the tunnels into the depths of the mine, the miners had carved small altars into the walls. In the deepest part of the mine, they had actually built a church. The link between religion and survival was apparent for all to see that far below the surface.

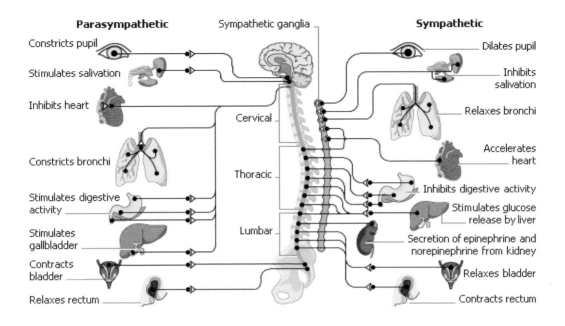

Parasympathetic		Sympathetic ganglia		Sympathetic
Constricts pupil				Dilates pupil
Stimulates salivation				Inhibits salivation
Inhibits heart		Cervical		Relaxes bronchi
Constricts bronchi				Accelerates heart
Stimulates digestive activity		Thoracic		Inhibits digestive activity
Stimulates gallbladder		Lumbar		Stimulates glucose release by liver
Contracts bladder				Secretion of epinephrine and norepinephrine from kidney
Relaxes rectum				Relaxes bladder
				Contracts rectum

The parasympathetic and sympathetic nervous systems and target organs.

Exercise and the Brain

I found it very interesting that the organization that was heavily involved in helping the miners and the Chilean government deal with the crisis was NASA. When the miners emerged from below the surface, they looked remarkably healthy. This is because they implemented specific techniques which NASA had learned from experiments developed in preparation for the isolation that astronauts would likely face during a Mars mission. For example, to combat the psychological stress, the miners set up an area for exercise. Each day, they walked back and forth in a small area of the tunnel. The exercise and limited caloric intake not only kept the miners lean so that they could fit in the escape capsule, but also had profound positive effects on their

TAKE A MOMENT TO RELAX BEFORE YOU EAT

If the sympathetic system is dominant, for example, during a stressful workday, then the digestive system is inhibited. This means that nutrients and fuels from the foods we eat during the day are not fully digested. So eating at your desk may make you feel like you're being productive, but the lack of necessary fuel and nutrients will have a negative effect on your performance in the afternoon. Most people experience a period of afternoon fatigue. Simply relaxing for a few moments before eating, and not working while eating, can make a big difference in your fuel and nutrient absorption. This is a critical reminder to add to your day to maximize your health and performance.

central and peripheral nervous systems. You could see these results in the physical and mental states of the miners when they were finally freed after months of ordeal.

The European Space Agency is conducting a study called Mars 500, where volunteers are completely isolated from the world for 500 days. They live in confined spaces which mimic the expected conditions in a spaceship that will travel from Earth to Mars. During the 500 days, the volunteers and scientists conduct experiments to study the effects of isolation on the human body and mind. One of the experiments involves the effects of exercise on the brain. The volunteers wear form-fitting caps with electrodes that measure brain activity (called electroencephalography [EEG]) and then take measurements before and after exercise. These results are not yet publicly available, but research on the effects of exercise on the brain is growing. Published studies on the use of new MRI technologies are helping us learn a great deal about the powerful effects of exercise on the brain.

Dr. Fred Gage from the Salk Institute for Biological Studies in La Jolla, California, has shown that exercise increases the volume of nerve tissue in the hippocampus in humans who exercise consistently over time.[19] The hippocampus is the area of the brain that is closely associated with the formation of memories and also the area specifically affected by aging. Dr. Gage and his research team have shown that exercise stimulates neurogenesis, or growth of new nerve cells and connections, in the dentate gyrus (the specific area in the hippocampus where new memories are formed). Interestingly, the dentate gyrus is also thought to be involved in depression and stress. Chronic stress has been shown to inhibit neurogenesis in the dentate gyrus, possibly as a result of increased stress hormones such as cortisol. Perhaps that is why people become forgetful when under constant stress. Clearly, the scientists at NASA did their research when consulting with the Chilean government on how best to help the miners deal with isolation and stress.

Perhaps the most exciting aspect of Dr. Gage's research was that the increases in the volume of the dentate gyrus in people who exercise correlated with improvements in cognitive function and cardiopulmonary fitness. There was a significant correlation between improvement in VO_{2max} (see Chapter 1) and increases in the volume of the dentate gyrus. Further, the research team, using the Rey Auditory Verbal Learning Test to measure recall, recognition and source memory, found that learning and delayed recall were improved after training and that the improvement in performance on the learning tests was related to the improvement in VO_{2max}. This relationship suggests that the greater the increase in fitness, the better the participants performed on their learning and memory tests. This finding is critical and should serve as a wake-up call to all the busy people whose jobs require a high degree of cognitive demand, but who are "too busy to go to the gym." And because the hippocampus is one of the brain areas subject to age-related decline, exercise may have a protective effect on the brain as we age. This subject is explored in detail in the wonderful book *Spark*, by Dr. John J. Ratey (www.johnratey.com/newsite/index.html).

Only a small percentage of Olympic athletes—fewer than 25%—will have lifetime best performances at the Olympics. During my master's degree research, I was able to take time to do background research on all the studies that examined Olympic athletes who performed well compared with those who did not. Some interesting conclusions emerged about the habits of the elite athletes who are high performers—and the answers reminded me of a famous quote by golf legend Arnold Palmer: "Golf is 90% mental, and the rest is in your head." Well, the same may be true for Olympians.

Let's begin with the end in mind, the final goal. And that is to perform at your best, to feel that relaxed energy, to enter the high-performance zone. I experienced this feeling only a few times in my swimming career. The most powerful moment was when I was attempting to qualify for the Olympic trials. I had broken my neck 14 months before the event, had undergone spinal reconstructive surgery and three months of rehab, and then trained like a maniac to get fit enough fast enough to have a chance to try out for the Olympics. I knew the split times I needed for my 200-metre backstroke, and had prepared and tapered perfectly. When I started the race I was amazed at how easy everything felt. It was almost as if my body was separated from my arms and legs. It was "fast/easy," not "fast/hard"—a critical distinction. When I look back on that moment, I remember one thing most clearly. I turned at the 100-metre mark and was able to see my splits on the race clock. I was not where I needed to be to qualify. Even though a great deal depended on my performance (I had suffered through a lot to get to this point), the only thought that went through my head when I saw the poor split time was "Hmm." Almost like "interesting." That's it. No panic, no fear, just recognition of where I was. Because of this reaction, I stayed relaxed. No tension entered my muscles or my mind. I simply increased my turnover, started to pick up my kicking earlier than I had planned, and swam faster than I ever had before in my life—even faster than before my accident. And I qualified for the Olympic trials. Although I did not make the team, I was proud to have had the chance to try out for it despite having fractured three vertebrae 16 months before. And it all happened because I was "in the zone" when it mattered the most.

Researchers have studied this concept of peak performance, or the zone. Unfortunately, attaining peak performance or entering the zone is still considered to be rare and involuntary. I don't believe that's true. If we can set the physiological stage with a great taper, then add in the psychological habits of successful Olympians, I think high performance becomes inevitable. In my research on this topic, I looked at the characteristics of peak performance described by those who had experienced it. They described being in complete control, experiencing effortless automatic performances, having a narrow focus of attention, being relaxed, feeling confident and having no fear of failure. My own experience seemed to fit right in with those research findings. So I knew I was on the right track, and the next step for me was to look at the reported differences between highly successful and less successful athletes in competition.

I found six research studies that had used psychological inventories to evaluate the characteristics of successful athletes at major games. All six reported that high self-confidence was a distinguishing factor between highly successful and less successful athletes. Other characteristics reported included (1) use of internal imagery more often (reported in five of the six studies); (2) lower anxiety/use of anxiety-control techniques more often (reported in four of the six studies); (3) use of positive self-talk more often (reported in three of the six studies); and (4) more focus and/or better concentration (reported in three of the six studies).

The interesting theme for me as a scientist engaged in helping athletes prepare for international competitions is that all these successful performers used different mental skills to achieve the same thing: to be able to focus on their performance while under pressure. This aim may seem simple, but under the magnifying glass of the Olympic Games it is not an easy thing to achieve. Needless to say, we all face equivalent challenges to perform, or struggle in our daily lives (although the pressure is much less). The skills and techniques that these athletes use with success at the Games will work for any of us in business, academics, music or personal relationships. When applied at the right moment, they can be powerful in helping us perform at our best.

Some world-class athletes are using an interesting technique called biofeedback and neurofeedback to train the nervous system to be able to perform under pressure. Penny Werthner, PhD, a professor at the University of Ottawa, a sports psychology consultant and a former Olympic athlete, has been using the assessment and training tool of biofeedback and neurofeedback with Olympic athletes and coaches since 2007. She conducted a three-year research program with the national freestyle ski team in preparation for the 2010 Winter Olympic Games in Vancouver, and is continuing this research with the national canoe kayak team leading up to the 2012 Olympic Games in London.

The findings from the three-year study indicated that all 10 athletes developed a greater level of awareness and regulation of the physiological and neurological responses under both stress and relaxation. Physiologically, they learned to enhance the regulation of the sympathetic/ parasympathetic balance of the autonomic nervous system to more efficiently manage their anxiety levels. Neurologically, they developed a greater awareness of the various mental states at work and the importance of developing the ability to shift those mental states (first step); and an actual ability to effectively shift mental states when needed (second step). The greatest improvement was in regulation of respiration rate, muscle tension and peripheral body temperature. The electrodermal response (arousal regulation) and heart-rate variability self-regulation ranges still required training to meet optimal levels, although considerable improvement was seen. All 10 athletes still needed work in sustaining their ideal focusing state and more quickly refocusing to that state when they became distracted. Two of the athletes in the three-year study won Olympic medals at the 2010 Vancouver Olympic Games.

Dr. Werthner has suggested that it's important to understand the link between physiological and psychological states. An athlete's ability to put himself or herself into an optimal focusing state within a stressful environment is closely related to the ability to let the body and mind relax and recover when appropriate. Two crucial components for success in high-performance sports are the ability to turn off the stress response, allowing parasympathetic dominance at will; and the ability to train the mind to shift states away from worry and rumination to either a narrow or a broad focus, depending on whether it's time to perform or not. The findings of this research can be used by both athletes and their coaches to assist in improving performance. As one athlete said, "Now I really get it when I need to be really focused; and all the rest of the time I can be breathing, resting, not focused." The question then becomes, "How do I relax and focus under pressure?" This is a question on the mind of almost all high performers in sports, music, academics and business.

Bio/neurofeedback training targets the development of an athlete's psychological skills of focus, anxiety management and recovery/relaxation ability to enhance overall sport performance. It involves the development of awareness and regulation of both physiological and neurological activity in the body and brain. Here are two techniques that you can practise by simply watching your heart rate or breathing rate.

In the first technique, Dr. Werthner used a photoplethysmyograph monitor on the non-dominant thumb, which gives an indirect measure of heart rate. Alternatively, you can use a simple heart-rate monitor, or take your pulse using your fingers. Typically, athletes show much lower-than-average heart rates, but genetics and conditioning determine the baseline. Heart-rate variability (HRV) refers to the rise and fall of the heart rate synchronized with each breath. The magnitude of this systemic variability reflects a healthy alternation between two autonomic influences on the heartbeat—the sympathetic and the parasympathetic. Lack of this variation reflects an imbalance between the two aspects of the autonomic nervous system (ANS), most likely due to a deficient parasympathetic influence. The variability of heart rate is what is of interest. The athlete observes the trace and uses it as feedback for regulating the breath and/or emotional state. Simply put, the more relaxed you are, the lower your heart rate and heart rate variability. The visual feedback from the equipment (or simply your pulse) can give you some feedback on how successful you are at relaxing mentally and physically.

The second technique is to use breathing as an indication of mental and physical relaxation. Respiration pattern, which means the depth and frequency of breathing, is highly sensitive to changes in arousal level and emotions. A shallow breathing pattern in athletes has been identified as one of the physiological indicators of stress. Diaphragmatic breathing reduces sympathetic arousal, a state that encourages regeneration, releases tension, and increases physical and mental relaxation. The instrument used to determine breathing frequency is a strain gauge around the abdomen below the rib cage. Deregulation in breathing often happens during tasks and is usually indicated by one or more of three variations: (1) shallow breathing, with the shoulders doing most of the work; (2) breath-holding during tasks; and (3) increasing respiration rate (breaths per minute). All three variations are associated with poor performance in sport and many other performance situations.

EXERCISE AND NERVOUS-SYSTEM HEALTH

It's not just the body that is improved by exercise. Health professionals are learning that exercise can help improve the brain function of people with a number of conditions. Researchers at the Tacoma family medicine program at the University of Washington have reported that exercise reduces the symptoms of depression as effectively as such traditional treatments as cognitive behaviour therapy or pharmacologic antidepressant therapy, and more effectively than bright-light therapy.[22] The researchers also report that combined strength and aerobic exercises are more effective than aerobic training alone, and that other methods, such as tai chi and yoga, also reduce the symptoms of depression. Given the complex neurobiology of depression, this new research does not mean anyone suffering from the condition should stop any therapies the doctor has prescribed. However, these studies suggest that exercise is another option that can be added to the treatment regimen of patients with symptoms of depression.

If exercise can change our nervous system for the better, the next question is, What is the best kind of exercise for achieving that goal? I was introduced to yoga by a good friend, Jody Holden, who was a member of

VISUALIZATION AND MENTAL REHEARSAL

Visualization and mental rehearsal are approaches to improving performance that involve the use of controlled "daydreams." These skills enable you to picture a comforting scene or to rehearse a performance task such as a race. Mental imagery can play a role in the learning of movements and the improvement of motor performance. Visualization causes the brain to release neurotransmitters that in turn help you to relax (decreased muscle tension), increase your energy (improved circulation of glycogen and oxygen) and resist disease (increased white blood-cell count). It's a powerful tool that can improve performance and health. Mental rehearsal—imagining a performance— can help you practise a performance before you do it. It can improve your memory, enhance your creativity and help you identify and solve problems.

Use images of	in order to
a relaxing scene	handle pressure and improve sleep
an energizing scene	increase motivation and excitement before a race
a successful past performance	help you enter a high-performance state of body and mind and improve your confidence

Method

Lean back, relax and practise your progressive relaxation routine.

Place your hand against your stomach. Inhale slowly through your nose for 4 seconds, feeling your abdomen expand. Exhale through your mouth for 8 seconds. Repeat.

Now picture a vivid scene that you associate with total relaxation (or energy, or success)—for example, a beach, cottage or other vacation spot. Make it as real and as detailed as possible. See the objects, patterns and colours all around you. Smell the smells, hear the sounds, and feel the sensations and temperatures.

Notice with each breath that you let go of tension, worries and problems, and that you enjoy being relaxed and happy in a very positive place.

Review your success, your positive reactions and your feelings of confidence, control, commitment and competence. Remind yourself that you can feel this way any time you wish.

Open your eyes, stand up and stretch.

You can practise these and other techniques on your own. Once you have the feeling of what it's like to control your mental and physical activation levels, you'll be able to control your thoughts when it matters most.

Canada's beach volleyball team. Jody and his partner, Conrad Leinemann, won a gold medal at the 1999 Pan Am Games and represented Canada at the Olympics in Sydney. Jody dragged me to class one day, and from that moment I was hooked. Yoga is the first exercise I've tried where I actually felt much

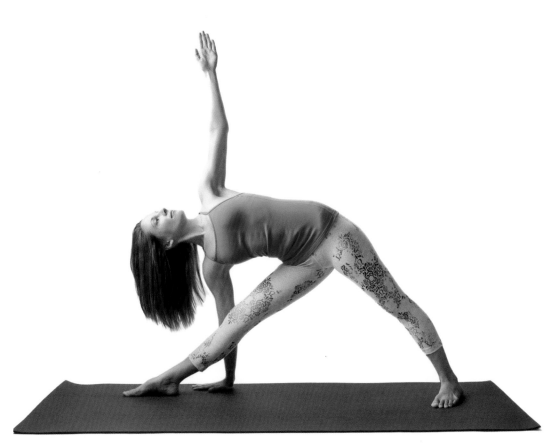

Yoga is useful for more than stress management. It strengthens the muscles and can even change the brain.

better right after the workout. Yoga has its roots in the Indus Valley of India, where a Hindu teacher named Patañjali recorded its first principles in religious scriptures known as the Yoga Sūtras. Modern varieties have emerged, and today nearly 20 million people practise yoga in North America.

Yoga has been the focus of intense research. Several papers have been published that show the powerful effect of yoga on neurotransmitters.[24] Yoga practice has been shown to increase melatonin production (see Chapter 7) as well as GABA, dopamine and serotonin levels, while lowering cortisol. Yoga also significantly decreases sympathetic

STRETCH TO STAY HEALTHY

Full-body stretching is an excellent activity that should be included in your daily routine. Stretching is a conscious lengthening of muscles to enhance flexibility and relieve joint pain. It's also a warm-up activity before rigorous exercise or sport. Scientists advise that stretching be done only after 5 to 10 minutes of warm-up or after a workout. It should never be performed when the muscles are cold. Ideally, an average person should stretch daily. Each stretch should last for just 1 or 2 seconds if loosening up before a workout, and 15 to 30 seconds if stretching after a workout or for relaxation.

Here are a few scientific benefits of stretching:

- ► reduced muscle tension and increased flexibility
- ► enhanced muscular coordination
- ► improved balance
- ► relief from muscle pain

- ► increased joint flexibility
- ► increased range of motion
- ► relaxation of tightened muscles and joints
- ► improved posture

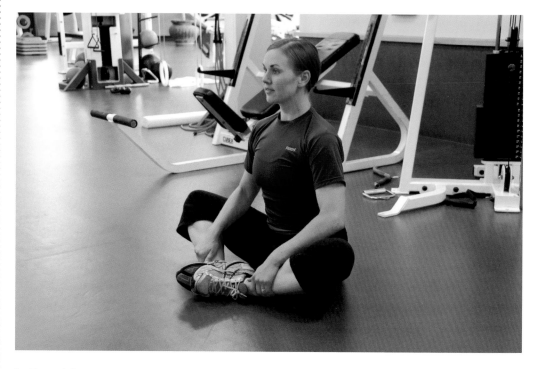

For this stretch, first sit comfortably with your legs out in front of you. Set your upper body with good posture and focus on keeping your spine straight and upright. Bringing together the insides of your feet, bend your knees and allow them to drop off to the side. Slowly draw your feet closer to your body. You should feel a stretch in the insides of your legs and your groin area. Breathe and try to let tension release from your body.

Overstretching can lead to ischemia, muscle rupture, weakened bones or even permanent damage to any part of your body. To avoid such injuries, it's important you understand some basic facts.

- ▶ Stretch only for 10 to 15 minutes and only when the muscles are warm.
- ▶ If you experience any kind of pain while stretching, it is advisable to stop immediately and consult a doctor.
- ▶ Breathe normally, taking in air through the nose and taking it out through the mouth.
- ▶ Try to take as much time as you need to complete your stretching process. Initial guidance on such exercises is essential.
- ▶ Do not lock your joints while stretching.

In this exercise, you can combine some core strengthening with flexibility. Standing tall and with a good posture, grasp a light bar in your hands. (Hands should be placed slightly wider apart than shoulder width.) Take your right foot and move it forward, slowly placing it in front and to the left of your left foot (see picture). Contract your abdominal muscles and slowly raise your arms and the bar over your head. Once the bar is directly overhead and you have control of your balance, slowly move the bar laterally to your left. Continue until you feel a stretch on the right side of your torso. (You may also feel this stretch on the outside of your right leg and hip.) Hold the position for a few seconds. Slowly return to an upright posture and then lower your arms and uncross your legs. Repeat to the other side.

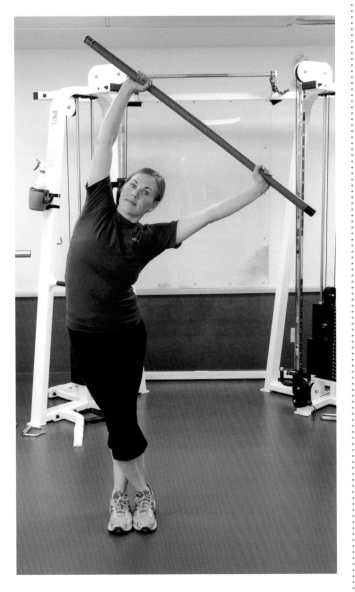

THE RELATIONSHIP BETWEEN EXERCISE AND MENTAL HEALTH

Researchers from Norway have published data showing exercising at any level is associated with better physical and mental health in men and women when compared with people who do not exercise. Interestingly, the relationship between exercise and mental health appears more pronounced in older individuals. So the older we get, the more powerful exercise becomes for keeping mentally healthy.

nervous system activity,[25] and thereby heart rate and blood pressure. After eight weeks of yoga practice, heart rate variability was shown to decrease—a sign that the sympathetic nervous system was more relaxed.

Amazingly, meditation may be even more powerful than yoga in its effects on the brain. Dr. Britta Hölzel from the Massachusetts General Hospital used MRI scans to look at the brains of 16 healthy people before and after they completed an eight-week meditation program.[26] None of the participants had practised meditation before the experiment, and the participants followed a common training technique called mindfulness-based stress reduction (MBSR). Anatomical images from the brains of the participants were compared with brain scans from 17 people who were on the waiting list for the study. The MRI images revealed that the meditation program increased grey matter in the left hippocampus, the posterior cingulate cortex, the temporo-parietal junction and the cerebellum. Remember, the hippocampus is an area of the brain closely associated with learning and memory, and the cerebellum is the area that serves to coordinate movements. The posterior cingulate cortex, a fascinating part of the brain that appears to be activated by emotional words,[27] may be an important structure for helping us relate to the beliefs of others. The temporo-parietal junction helps us distinguish between ourselves and others, and is involved specifically in reasoning about the contents of another person's mind as well as understanding others.[28] Damage to this area has been associated with out-of-body experiences and impaired moral judgment. Each of these important areas of the brain was positively affected by the meditation training. So think about incorporating meditation—even for a few minutes—into your daily routine.

Given today's environment of high pressure and stress, meditation and yoga seem to be perfect activities to help us recover from intense work and keep us healthy. I currently recommend that the athletes and corporate clients I work with try to do one or two yoga sessions a week. I encourage them to try various styles of yoga until they find a teacher and style they enjoy. Many people recommend that meditation be practised daily. As little as five minutes a day can help calm the mind, relax the body and reduce stress and anxiety. For more information on meditation, consider reading *Meditation: The First and Last Freedom*, by Osho.

NUTRITION AND THE NERVOUS SYSTEM

Did you know that what you eat affects the way you feel, your mood and your energy levels? You may be intuitively aware of this connection, but research now substantiates what many people, including medical professionals, have been saying for years. Tragically, the Western diet is devoid of many of the nutrients that we need for the proper functioning of the nervous system. Nutrient deficiencies and diet in general may play a role in nervous system diseases such as anxiety and depression. The health benefits of the Mediterranean diet, which are well known and widely accepted, are mostly related to lower risk of cardiovascular disease and cancer, and longer life expectancy when compared with other populations. But there's also significant evidence that foods can have a powerful effect on the nervous system.

Recently, a significant body of research has brought to light the powerful effects of foods and nutrients on mental health, and specifically depression.[29] People with diets that are high in fish, fruits and vegetables have protection against the symptoms of depression, whereas those whose diets are high in processed meat, milk chocolate (dark chocolate that is above 80% cocoa is actually quite good for you in small amounts), sweet desserts, fried food, refined cereal and high-fat dairy have increased vulnerability to depression. These findings have been shown in large sample sizes in Britain[30] (3486 people) and Spain[31] (10,094 people), among other places. These studies suggest an inverse relationship between the incidence of depression in the population and the intake of fruits and nuts, mono-unsaturated fats such as olive oil, and legumes. A lack of B-vitamins, iron, zinc, magnesium, chromium, vitamin D and omega-3 fatty acids has been shown to be specifically related to depression—and these nutrients have been used as part of treatment programs for the

GREG'S HIGH-PERFORMANCE TIPS

THE MEDITERRANEAN DIET IS YOUR BEST CHOICE

The Mediterranean diet is characterized by an emphasis on vegetables, fresh and dried fruits, whole-grain cereals, nuts and legumes, olive oil and a moderate amount of red wine. Foods are high in antioxidants, magnesium, zinc and other micronutrients. The main protein source in the diet is fish, with some meat and dairy included. The diet is also very high in omega-3 fatty acids.

BREAKFAST OF CHAMPIONS

There are several examples of how tryptophan and tyrosine levels can influence mental health and performance in times of war, both for civilians and for soldiers. The round-the-clock bombing in Iraq during the prelude to the Desert Storm invasion—the "Shock and Awe" campaign—had a physiological rationale. The constant stress that the population and the military experienced during this phase of the campaign would have resulted in the constant activation of the central nervous system, and the sympathetic nervous system specifically. Tyrosine is a precursor for (it is used to build) the neurotransmitters dopamine, epinephrine and norepinephrine. After a period of constant stress, such as during the bombing of Baghdad, the neurons of the brain were likely working constantly to pump out these neurotransmitters. After some time, the demand for the neurotransmitters would have exceeded the supply of tyrosine from proteins that were eaten during that time. The objective of the bombing, therefore, may not have been to destroy physical targets, but to deplete the population and military staff of essential neurotransmitters. This depletion would have caused people to develop behavioural and cognitive problems. Specifically, there would have been increases in depression, lethargy, and memory and attention control.

illness. Depression is a very complicated condition; nutrition likely plays a key role in the prevention and management of this disease, but should be considered only as a component of a comprehensive treatment plan implemented under the supervision of a medical professional.

The implications of the relationship between nutrients and conditions that negatively affect the brain and its function are profound. If we can gain control of our psychological health and mood by using nutrition, then improved health and performance can be controlled rather than be a random outcome of our daily lives and habits. Specifically, the foods we eat can have an impact on our alertness and our relaxation. The reason behind this is that neurotransmitters—the chemicals that the nerves in our brain, spinal cord and peripheral nervous system use to communicate—are made up of amino acids. Amino acids are the components that make up proteins. The amino acid tyrosine has been shown to help increase the levels of the "alertness" neurotransmitters dopamine and norepinephrine; and tryptophan has been shown to increase the production of serotonin, a neurotransmitter that helps relax the brain. According to Trionne Moore, who as lead nutritionist for the Canadian Sport Centre in Toronto works extensively with Olympic athletes, "A breakfast with the right balance of both stimulating and calming foods starts a person off with a brain that is primed to learn and emotions in control. Eating complex carbohydrates along with proteins helps to usher the amino acids from these proteins into the brain, so that the neurotransmitters can work better."

Knowing this, scientists from the Naval Aerospace Research Laboratory in Pensacola, Florida, have conducted a study on the use of tyrosine as a countermeasure to prevent decreases in performance among soldiers during sustained military operations. Soldiers often face continuous work periods that last longer than 12 hours (often for many days at a time). There may not be time to sleep, and they suffer from extreme fatigue. This may sound typical of many people in North America, so the applications of this research likely extend beyond the military. Military scientists have experimented with supplemental tyrosine (which is also found in protein-rich foods) and have found that it preserves levels of norepinephrine in the brains of stressed animals. It also prevents decrements in performance in humans who are exposed to extended periods of stress.[32] Tyrosine supplementation also appears to prevent the rise in cortisol that accompanies stressful events. Research in this area is ongoing, but I do suggest that people who have to perform under stress or at high intensities for extended periods consume foods that have a high protein-to-carbohydrate ratio. Examples include such protein-rich foods as meat, poultry, seafood, beans, tofu and lentils matched with complex carbohydrates such as whole grains or brown/wild rice.

HEALTHY FOOD OPTIONS FOR A HEALTHY BRAIN

Specific foods are extremely beneficial for improving and nurturing brain function. Complex carbohydrates, vitamin C, vitamin E, omega-3 fatty acids, folic acid, vitamins B12 and B6, antioxidant nutrients and beta-carotene are the nutrients that will enhance the functioning of the brain. Below is a list of foods which can contribute to a healthy brain and nervous system.

Foods that contain omega-3 fatty acids, including fish, are beneficial for effective functioning of the brain. Wild salmon, tuna and mackerel are excellent sources of essential fats. Tuna is also rich in vitamin B (niacin), which protects our brain from Alzheimer's disease. Egg yolk is an excellent source of choline. Choline is made up of two fat-like molecules that are present in the brain. Kidney beans are rich in inositol, which may help in improving depression and mood disorders. Inositol is a part of the B-complex vitamin family. Researchers have found that one cup of kidney beans contains almost 19% of the recommended daily value for the B-vitamin thiamin. Olive oil contains a good amount of omega-3 fatty acids. Honey contains antioxidants, which protect the cells from damage caused by free radicals. Nuts, among the healthiest snacks, are rich in zinc, which is essential for maintaining the nervous system. Blueberries, cranberries and strawberries contain antioxidants. Wheat germ is a powerful brain food rich in selenium, vitamin E, magnesium and choline. Sweet potatoes contain vitamin C and beta-carotene, which act as antioxidant nutrients. Sweet potatoes are an excellent source of vitamin B6, which is necessary for the manufacturing of neurotransmitters.

Where tyrosine appears to help increase focus, mental performance and resistance to stress, the amino acid tryptophan has quite different effects. The high concentration of tryptophan can increase its uptake into the brain, where it's used to synthesize the brain neurotransmitter 5-hydroxytryptamine, also known as serotonin (5-HT). There is significant evidence that 5-HT is involved in central fatigue, or the way the brain controls our mental and physical sensations of fatigue. 5HT release is associated with sleep and drowsiness, which means that eating foods that are high in tryptophan, along with carbohydrates, is an excellent option late in the day if you're trying to calm down and prepare for sleep.

Foods can have powerful effects on the brain's neurotransmitter levels, and thus on our moods and mental capacities. But what about exercise performance? The concept of central fatigue, where the brain controls fatigue during exercise, is the topic of intense research and controversy. Perhaps the best example is the recent study from the School of Sport and Exercise Sciences at the University of Birmingham.[33] The researchers found that a simple rinse with a drink high in sugars increases exercise performance, even though the cyclists who were tested did not actually swallow any of the drink. The findings suggest that the brain can sense nutrients that it *expects* should be arriving in the stomach, intestines, blood and then muscles, and thus keeps the exercise going at a high level—even though the expected sugar boost never arrives in the stomach. The scientists at the University of Birmingham followed up the exercise study with MRI neuro-imaging studies and found that rinsing the mouth with carbohydrate solutions activated the insula/frontal operculum, orbitofrontal cortex and striatum. These areas of the brain are believed to be involved in reward and motor control. Simply stimulating these areas of the brain with a glucose solution in the mouth improved endurance exercise performance. These findings in no way mean that the brain is always responsible for the perception of fatigue, but they do provide some strong evidence that the brain is closely involved in the regulation of exercise performance.

The brain, spinal cord and peripheral nerves are the control system for the entire body. An understanding of how our nervous system works and how it can become fatigued can help all of us appreciate the amazing achievements of world-class performers. It also explains why we get tired after long days at work and why learning to maintain focus is so critical (and hard). Ultimately, it explains how to unlock the potential of our minds and bodies. The brain is an organ that needs to be fuelled and exercised, just like our muscles. A better understanding of the nervous system will lead to techniques we can implement in our day-to-day lives to improve our health and performance. The exciting new information about the brain and nervous system has the potential to revolutionize our health and performance. By applying some of the nutrition and exercise tips in this chapter you can take steps toward optimizing the health of your nervous system and improving your performance at work, enhancing the activities that you are passionate about.

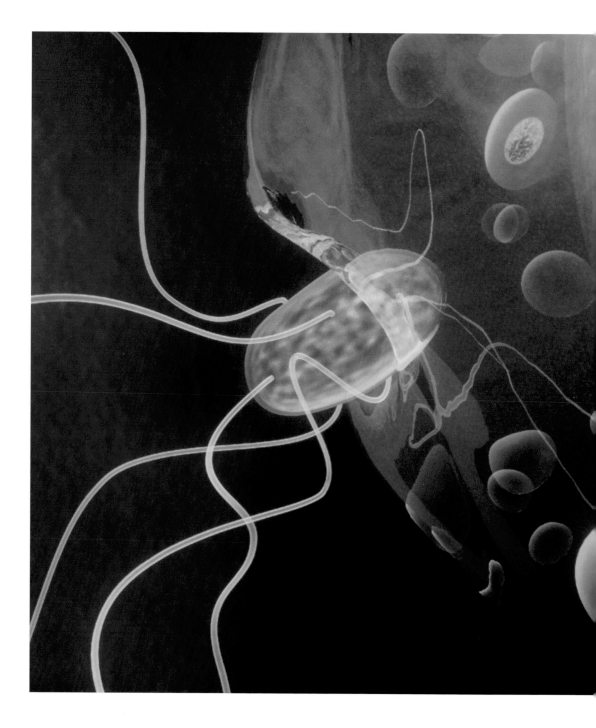

RESISTING ILLNESS AND DISEASE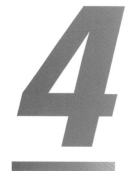

The Immune System

Most international-level athletes train 20 to 30 hours a week over 10 or more years for a chance to compete on the world's stage. Imagine you've trained tirelessly for more than a decade. You've thought of everything and prepared endlessly to make sure you have the best chance of reaching your potential. Then, on the plane to your event, you pick up a virus and get sick. Even an infection as simple as the common cold can disrupt your performance and end your dreams. Of course, a cold makes the rest of us feel awful, too; we miss work, and our day-to-day activities suffer. Maintaining health is so important that, over the past 20 years, exercise immunology has become a new field of interest. Great advances are being made in our knowledge of how to keep athletes healthy during stressful training, through intense competition, and while travelling. Of course, the great thing about this new knowledge, as it relates to athletes, is that we, the general public, can benefit from it. We can apply these techniques to keep ourselves healthier. In this chapter, I'll show you how the immune system works; why we experience colds, flus, fevers and infections; and how we can use exercise to improve the immune system and our overall health.

UNDERSTANDING THE EXERCISE–IMMUNITY RELATIONSHIP

A fascinating paradox in human physiology is the concept of a J-shaped relationship between exercise training and health. The "J-shaped hypothesis" suggests that, in general, people who exercise regularly experience fewer illnesses and infections than those who do not. The relationship is based on research that measured the number of upper

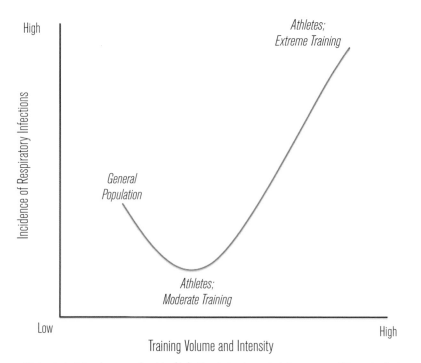

High

Incidence of Respiratory Infections

Athletes;
Extreme Training

General
Population

Athletes;
Moderate Training

Low

High

Training Volume and Intensity

Moderate training decreases the risk of infection, but extreme training or competition actually increases it.

respiratory tract infections (URTIs), such as the common cold, that people experience every year. Although this relationship was developed based on the incidence of URTIs, more recent studies have explored the relationship between exercise and other diseases. They have found that exercise affords protection against many diseases, even cancer. However, increasing the amount of exercise beyond moderate levels does not improve immunity further. Quite the opposite happens. When athletes train at volumes and intensities excessively higher than normal for extended periods, they experience a significant increase in illnesses, as you can see in the figure above.

A published series of experiments highlights this relationship quite clearly. In the first experiment,[34] a group of mice were divided into two groups. One group rested in their cages, and the other ran to exhaustion for about 120 minutes for three consecutive days. Then both groups were exposed to a flu virus. Those who had exercised became sick earlier and had more severe symptoms. In the second experiment, mice were divided into three groups. The first group rested, the second group exercised at moderate intensity for 20 to 30 minutes, and the third group exercised to exhaustion. The J-shaped relationship was clearly evident: 50% of the sedentary mice, 12% of the moderate exercisers and 70% of the heavy exercisers experienced flu symptoms.

Research suggests that this relationship is also true for humans. A recent study followed a group of physically active adults over the fall and winter months. The researchers found those adults who exercised more than five days a week at a low to moderate intensity experienced cold symptoms for half the number of days that their less active counterparts did. Furthermore, the severity of symptoms was lower in the people who were the fittest.[35] This research provides yet another example of the benefits of exercise for the general population—increase your activity levels to a moderate amount, about five or six hours each week—and you can expect to experience fewer illnesses over the course of the year.

At the high end of the J-shaped relationship we can see that periods of very high intensity training, and by extension periods of high stress, are likely to increase the number and severity of upper respiratory tract infections. This observation suggests that the immune system may be impaired by very high intensity training or high levels of stress. From a scientific perspective, this impairment is possible. Dr. David Nieman from Appalachian State University in North Carolina has discovered that single bouts of high-intensity exercise, in this case a marathon, can cause a decrease in our natural killer cell activity, exposing us to greater risk of infection.[36] Dr. David Pyne from the Australian Institute for Sport has reported that long-term intense training may decrease the body's production of immunoglobulins that are secreted in our digestive and respiratory tracts, also causing an increased risk of infection.[37] Dr. Pyne's research was echoed in a recent paper by a research group from the University of São Paulo in Brazil. In that study, scientists looked at levels of immunoglobulin in the saliva of elite soccer players before and after a 70-minute match.[38] There was a significant decrease in salivary immunoglobulin A (IgA) after the match. Interestingly, the decrease was correlated with the perceived level of intensity of the match. In other words, the harder the players *thought* the game was, the worse their immune response after the game.

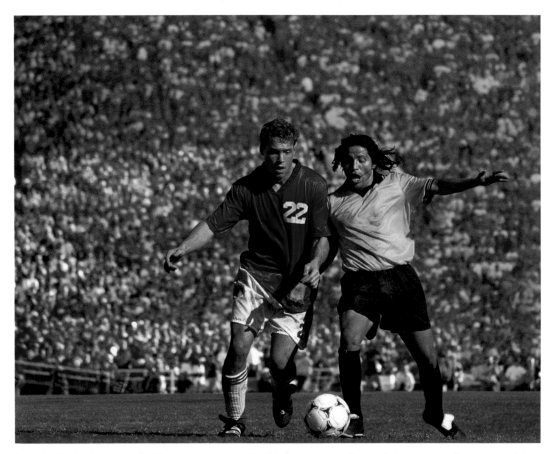

Immediately after intense exercise like a soccer game, an athlete's immune system is depressed, since energy and resources are being spent on refuelling and regenerating the body rather than defending it from invaders. After a workout, make sure to stay warm, wash your hands and avoid touching your eyes or mouth.

This immune suppression is temporary and may last from a few hours to a few days, depending on the volume and intensity of the exercise. It is sometimes referred to as the "open window." In this situation, a lower immunoglobulin level presents an opportunity for pathogens to gain access to the body. Immunoglobulins, also known as antibodies, are proteins produced by white blood cells that identify specific pathogens. Each immunoglobulin has the same basic structure, but with slightly different "tips" on the end of its protein chains—an analogy for this would be that you can change the head on a screwdriver to use it with different-sized objects. These different tips are specific to each invader encountered in the past. They allow the immunoglobulin to attach itself to and identify the invader so the immune system can mount a response and destroy the pathogen. The research paper on soccer players suggests that exhaustive exercise may cause a temporary suppression of these antibodies, creating a short-term open window where viruses, bacteria or other microbes may be able to access the body.

Athletes are under tremendous physical and mental stress. Most are intuitively aware of the J-shaped relationship, even if they have not read the research. Perhaps this is why so many turn to nutritional supplements in an effort to enhance immune function. Estimates of athletes who take some form of nutritional supplement range from about 20 to 80%, and research backs them up. It has shown that some supplements can improve muscle repair and help the immune system. It has been suggested that an amino acid called L-glutamine is used by the body to repair muscle tissue. Amino acids are structures that link together to make up proteins. L-glutamine is also used to fuel white blood cells: the lymphocytes, macrophages and fibroblasts. So when we train at a high level and cause micro-damage to the muscles, any L-glutamine that we eat in the form of proteins gets used to repair our muscles. Unfortunately, this may result in less L-glutamine being available for rebuilding white blood cells, thus increasing the chances of getting sick. Some people debate this rationale because research on the effect of up to two hours of exercise has not been shown to deplete the body's glutamine pool. [39] However, there is little research on the effects of training for more than two hours a day, or on what happens to glutamine levels while athletes are involved in high-intensity training camps and competition. So during training camps or periods of increased physical stress, it may still be helpful for athletes to supplement their diets with specific amino acids such as L-glutamine to provide their bodies with the nutrients needed for repairing muscles as well as keeping immune systems as strong as possible. Fortunately, most protein powders contain L-glutamine—just check the label. It is very important to note that, with L-glutamine and most other supplements, more is not necessarily better. L-glutamine is closely related to glutamate, a brain excitatory neurotransmitter. So overdosing on L-glutamine may have a negative impact on brain neurotransmitter levels.

> ## GREG'S HIGH-PERFORMANCE TIPS
> ### BOOSTERS FOR THE IMMUNE SYSTEM
> Psychological research from Wilkes University in Pennsylvania has demonstrated that levels of immunoglobulin A (the body's first line of defence against pathogens) is increased by up to 30% for several hours following intercourse.

Most research to date suggests that L-glutamine at doses of up to 3000 mg/day appears to be safe.

When we exercise, our breathing increases and provides our muscles with enough oxygen for mitochondria to convert our foods into energy. This energy then fuels our muscles' contractions during exercise. However, when oxygen is used by the body, by-products called reactive oxygen species (ROS) and free radicals are created. These reactive oxygen species and free radicals may decrease the locomotion and bactericidal abilities of white blood cells. Furthermore, they may decrease the proliferation of lymphocytes and inhibit natural killer cell activity levels.[40] Perhaps this is why there appears to be an "open window" when the immune system is compromised for a few hours after a very hard exercise session. To help protect yourself against free radical–induced impairment of the immune system after intense exercise, I suggest you take an antioxidant supplement containing vitamin C, vitamin E and beta-carotene. Of course, eating foods that are high in these nutrients is ideal, but supplements can help ensure you're getting what you need to keep yourself healthy during training or periods of high stress. Selenium is another antioxidant closely related to immune system function, but supplementing with selenium should be done with caution. Although amounts up to the recommended daily allowance have not been shown to have side effects, very high doses may cause some nausea and fatigue. Fruits and vegetables as well as whole grains and nuts are all high in antioxidants.

THE RELATIONSHIP BETWEEN TRAINING AND INFECTION

When athletes do get ill, the effects may devastate their performance. Former national team swimmer Dr. Thomas Zochowski and I have completed research that highlights this point. The influenza virus is an infection that is, unfortunately, well known. In 2009, the world became aware of a new strain called H1N1. Six weeks after a competitive swimmer in our monitoring program performed an incremental exercise, he was infected with H1N1. As I mentioned at the beginning of this chapter, when athletes catch a cold or get the flu it can be a major problem. They have to miss training and, for the duration of the infection, make no progress toward their goals. To make matters worse, some strains of the flu target muscle tissue as well as the respiratory tract, causing myositis (muscle inflammation). Our test results clearly demonstrated just how problematic getting sick is for an athlete.

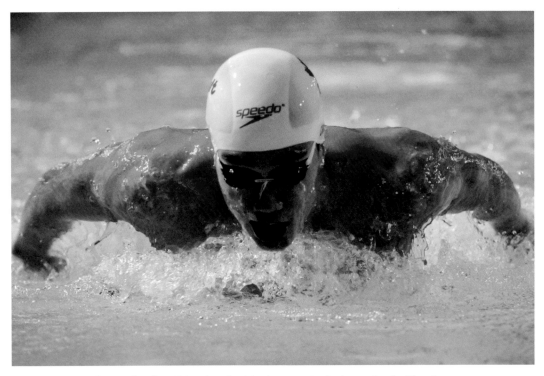

Double Olympian and Harvard graduate Tobias Oriwol training in preparation for the 2012 London Olympics.

In the exercise test, we evaluated the physiological responses (heart rate, in this case) to swimming at different speeds, from slow to very fast. An elevated resting heart rate is often seen before, during and after an infection because of the increased activity of the nervous system. In the case of the athlete who got sick, our testing showed that after the infection his heart rate was much higher than it would normally be. His heart rate was much higher at slower swimming speeds, reflecting increased activation of the sympathetic nervous system. Normally after extensive training, changes in the body make it easier to swim faster, thus lowering the heart rate at any given speed, reflecting that the athlete is in better condition, or has better technique, or is experiencing less stress on the nervous system than when the training began.

When he tried to go faster, the swimmer with H1N1 had only a slight increase in heart rate; moreover, he could not swim as quickly as he did in the previous test. It was as if his body had put a speed cap on his system to protect itself. It seems likely that the myositis caused by the H1N1 infection impaired his muscles' ability. Of course, the swimmer could also have

HERBS MAY HELP RESIST DISEASE
BUT MORE RESEARCH IS NEEDED

Herbal remedies are also often used to help reduce the duration and severity of upper respiratory tract infections, with Echinacea a popular choice. There are wide-ranging differences in the results of various studies, so we can't say for sure that Echinacea helps, although some research suggests it may work. It appears that Echinacea, taken after the onset of symptoms, does confer some benefit in terms of shortening the duration of the infection. Long-term supplementation, however, does not seem to help. Ginseng is another popular herb, especially with athletes. There is some evidence that ginseng helps to reduce fatigue and may have some immune-stimulating activity. The research on ginseng is not conclusive, although more studies are being published that should help to determine if it can help people with infections.

Sources: Block and Mead, 2003 [41]; Linde et al., 2006.[42]

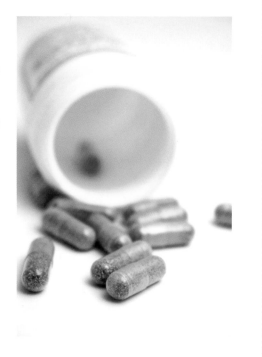

been experiencing some detraining and residual fatigue. We saw the same patterns in his blood lactate analysis, meaning that his anaerobic system was also affected by the infection.

CHANGES IN THE IMMUNE SYSTEM WHEN ATHLETES PREPARE FOR COMPETITION

When we rest or reduce our physical training load after a period of increased work (as when athletes "taper" before competition), the body responds by producing more of a specific blood cell called eosinophils. Eosinophils are white blood cells believed to detoxify some of the inflammation-inducing substances in the body. They destroy allergen-antibody complexes, thus preventing the spread of inflammation. Lymphocytes, another kind of white blood cell that fights infection, are also shown to increase during the taper phase leading into competitions. Normally, these physiological markers would be considered a sign the body is fighting an infection, but during taper the body may be responding to the reduced stress load by cleaning up all the damaged tissues. The increases in these cell counts that occur during taper are related to the reduction in training volume, so the more that training is reduced, the greater the number of lymphocytes that is produced.[43] A bonus of this hyperactivation of the immune system is that the body's capacity to resist illness improves during taper. That's good, because a cold is the last thing an athlete wants right before the Olympics. This relationship also applies to the general population and is why rest is so critical when we're starting to feel ill or are stressed out or injured. We are simply tapering the overall physical or mental stress that the body is under so that energy can be applied to the immune system to help fight off invaders or to heal damaged structures in the body. If you're starting to feel ill or stressed out, get some rest so you don't get sick.

ENVIRONMENTAL THREATS TO OUR HEALTH

Our environment is full of viruses, bacteria, microbes, toxins, parasites and other pathogens that constantly try to invade our bodies. The complex series of interconnected structures and organs that help us fight off these invaders is called the immune system.

To give you an idea of just how important the immune system is, consider that when we die and our immune system stops fighting off the pathogens that surround us, our bodies are invaded within minutes. The invaders break down the tissues of our bodies, and we decay and dissolve in a matter of days or weeks, depending on the environment. For example,

The key components of the immune system: the bones, the thymus gland and the lymphatic system. Bones create white blood cells. The thymus and the lymphatic system filter the blood.

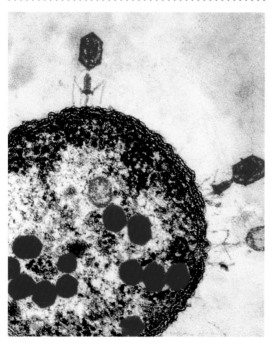

An electron micrograph of a virus latching on to a cell wall.

bodies decay quickly in the hot jungle but are preserved indefinitely near the top of an icy mountain. This concept was the foundation of H.G. Wells' famous book *The War of the Worlds*, written in 1898. It's the first novel to describe the invasion of Earth by Martians. The Martians successfully take over the world, and have no problem disposing of the human military resistance. However, they eventually succumb to pathogenic bacteria and all die. Although this story is a work of fiction, the view of our immune system as saving humans from destruction is absolutely true and relevant in our non-fiction world. It's amazing that our immune system is so powerful and capable of resisting this constant assault—keeping us healthy throughout our lives.

Our body's main enemies are viruses, bacteria, microbes and fungal infections. They are often collectively referred to as "germs." Bacteria are tiny single-cell organisms, most of them less than 1/100th the size of one of the body's 100 trillion cells. Each bacterium has a nucleus, organelles for producing energy, DNA and other cellular structures, and can eat and reproduce. This is what makes them dangerous—they feed on elements in our bodies that we need for health, and their waste products can be toxic. Bacteria reproduce very quickly, sometimes as fast as every 20 minutes. A single bacterium can become millions very quickly. However, some bacteria are beneficial. Our digestive tract has millions of bacteria that help digest food, and without them we can become quite sick. The challenge for our immune system therefore is to determine which bacteria are good for us and which are dangerous, and then eliminate the dangerous ones as quickly as possible. In most cases, the immune system is effective at targeting and destroying

DOES VITAMIN C IMPROVE IMMUNE HEALTH?

How to treat the common cold, and specifically the use of vitamin C to do so, has been a source of controversy for decades. In a recent review by Dr. Robert M. Douglas and Dr. Harri Hemilä , the impact of vitamin C supplementation in preventing and treating the common cold has been considerably clarified. The scientists looked at the results from 31 studies that included 11,350 participants to determine whether supplementing the diet with more than 0.2 grams per day of vitamin C decreased the incidence of colds. Their research showed that supplementing with vitamin C did not decrease the incidence of colds, but it did reduce the duration of cold symptoms by 8% in adults and 14% in children. Consistent supplementation appears to be the key.

Dr. Douglas and Dr. Hemilä also looked at studies of elite athletes and determined that in those participating in physically stressful events such as marathon running, cross-country skiing or physical training, vitamin C supplementation decreased the risk of infection by 50%. They also noted that one study, which had a very large sample size, indicated that treatment of the common cold with 8 grams of vitamin C per day after the onset of symptoms had a beneficial effect on the symptoms experienced. So, although I am sure there will be more research and debate on this topic, for now it appears that you should be taking some vitamin C regularly—and that you should increase the amount you take if you get a cold or participate in some serious physical activity. Excellent food sources of vitamin C include broccoli, bell peppers, kale, cauliflower, strawberries, lemons, mustard and turnip greens, Brussels sprouts, papaya, chard, cabbage, spinach, kiwi, snow peas, cantaloupe, oranges, grapefruit, limes, tomatoes, zucchini, raspberries, asparagus, celery, pineapple, lettuce, watermelon and fennel.[44]

bacterial invaders. But sometimes it needs help, and that is what antibiotics are designed for. Antibiotics have helped us overcome severe diseases such as polio, which is caused by bacteria that attack the nervous system and can leave us paralyzed. Another common bacterial infection is strep throat, which also can be treated by antibiotics.

Viruses are another common cause of infection in the human body. They are very different from bacteria in that they are not technically alive. Viruses are fragments of DNA in protective shells that invade host cells and start replicating, often destroying the host cell in the process. When a virus attacks a cell, the shell casing of the virus contacts the cell membrane and injects the virus's DNA into the cell. The viral DNA uses the existing machinery inside the host cell to replicate. When the cell dies, it releases the replicated viruses into the surrounding tissues. Not all viruses kill the host cell; some are able to hijack it and convert it into a virus factory. These manufactured viruses then escape the cell to circulate through the body and invade other cells. Viruses are the cause of many illnesses. For example, the rhinovirus causes the common cold, which affects the upper airways; the influenza virus causes the flu; the herpes simplex causes mumps; and the measles viruses can cause meningitis, which attacks the brain or spinal cord. HIV, the human immune deficiency virus, attacks the body's immune system itself.

In recent years, the treatment of viral infections has progressed immensely, and a new class of drugs called anti-retrovirals holds great promise for the future. These drugs work by interfering with the replication of viruses. However, more progress remains to be made because each drug must be highly specific to a target virus, and, like bacteria, viruses can develop resistance to these drugs. Unfortunately, viral infections still remain very difficult to treat. The body's immune system is therefore our primary mechanism of defence against these and other pathogens.

THE IMMUNE SYSTEM

The immune system is made up of tissues and blood cells that fight off invaders from the external environment. Our first line of defence against bacteria, viruses and other pathogens is the skin. The skin forms a barrier between our bodies and the environment, and is quite hostile to microbes. Microbes prefer an acidity similar to the internal environment of the human body, a pH of around 7. The pH of the skin is typically much lower, often less than 5. This acidic environment kills most of the microbes that come into contact with the skin, as long as the skin remains intact. This is why it's so important to keep skin wounds and cuts clean; if you don't, bacteria or other pathogens can gain access to deeper layers of the skin or even the bloodstream, causing infections that will require treatment with medications.

You can actually see the immune system at work when you get a cut or a splinter. Initially, you'll observe the cut bleeding. Blood contains elements called platelets that coagulate and clog the breaks in the skin to stop the bleeding. After this, there may be an invasion of bacteria and viruses from the cut, or from a foreign object such as a piece of wood if you have a splinter. The body identifies these invaders as foreign and mounts an all-out attack. What you see is the area becoming red and swollen. This inflammatory response arises because of the body's efforts to clean the wound, disinfect the area and heal the tissue.

After the skin, the most likely point of entry for a pathogen is the digestive tract, which your immune system also defends. We eat hundreds if not thousands of germs (bacteria, viruses, toxins or microbes) every day. Most of the time, the enzymes and acids of the digestive tract (stomach acids

SUPERBODIES

112

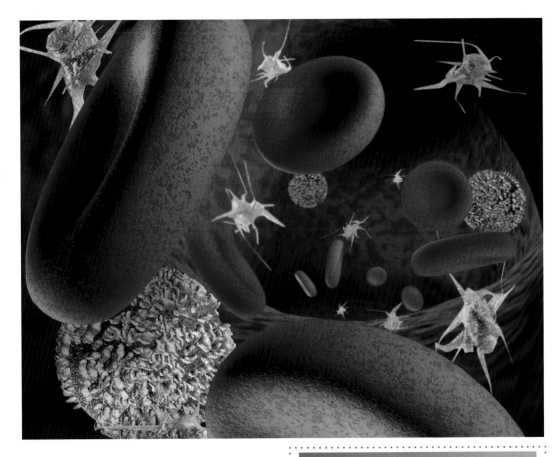

The view from just under the surface of the skin looking out through a cut. You can see the red blood cells, white blood cells, platelets and filaments—all components that will eventually close and heal the cut.

> ### 🏅 GREG'S HIGH-PERFORMANCE TIPS
>
> #### SUPERFOOD BOOSTERS FOR THE IMMUNE SYSTEM
>
> Superfoods that boost the immune system are ones that include vitamins A, B6, B12, C, D and E as well as folic acid, iron, zinc, copper and selenium.

have a pH of less than 2) deal with these germs and we're never aware of a problem. However, all it takes is one of these invaders to penetrate our defences for us to have food poisoning, and we'll definitely notice that. The symptoms of an infection of the digestive tract are usually vomiting and diarrhea. While most of us have few if any problems when at home, travelling to new destinations often exposes us to new bacteria and other types of germs in the water or foods. Anyone who has experienced stomach problems during a visit to a developing country can attest to this predicament.

Once the pathogen invaders make it past our initial defences, the job

113

CARBOHYDRATES FUEL OUR IMMUNE SYSTEM CELLS

Phagocytes consume glucose at a rate 10 times higher than they consume glutamine. Phagocytes are the macrophages (cells that literally eat or absorb other cells or foreign particles) that engulf invaders and then destroy them by breaking them up and literally digesting them. This process consumes energy, and the cells need fuel—in this case, glucose. To maintain blood-glucose levels, carbohydrates are very important. Therefore, we all need to pay attention to eating quality complex carbohydrates, especially when we're not feeling well. Complex carbohydrates are present in whole grain products, rice (but not white rice—go for wild or brown rice) and other foods that are high in fibre.[45]

ZINC IMPROVES LYMPHOCYTE FUNCTION

Zinc is a nutrient that's closely related to immune function.[46] Zinc deficiency has been shown to impair lymphocyte and phagocyte function, and a slight excess of zinc intake beyond the recommended daily allowance (currently at 8 to 11 mg /day for adults) may improve immune function. But again, more is not necessarily better, because taking zinc or any other vitamin or mineral above a certain threshold may actually reduce immune function.

of finding and destroying them is taken on by the cellular components of our immune system. In most cases, this job falls to the white blood cells—the body's professional assassins—which are produced in the bone marrow.

Many blood cells are produced in the bone marrow. White blood cells are the primary cells that fight foreign particles, bacteria and viruses throughout the body. The technical name for white blood cells is leukocytes; if you're looking at blood test results, this is the term you will see. Sixteen different kinds of white blood cells perform slightly different roles. Macrophages and neutrophils kill by ingesting microorganisms and then exposing the ingested materials to toxic chemicals or acids. Other kinds of white blood cells include natural killer cells and eosinophils that destroy invaders or damaged tissues on contact using chemicals. Simply put, some white blood cells absorb invaders to kill them; others kill them externally. We have many white blood cells in our blood— almost 5 billion per litre. White blood cells are slightly different from most other cells in the body; they are able to move on their own and so capture and destroy invaders.

Many white blood cells begin as stem cells. Once released into the bloodstream, stem cells change into different kinds of white blood cells, depending on what tissue they are in and the role they must play. For example, in lung tissue, stem cells turn into macrophages. Macrophages keep the lungs clean by absorbing and destroying pollution particles, dust or bacterial invaders. They are also present in the skin, where they are called Langerhans cells, and in the blood, where they swim around and help clean up injured tissue.

Other kinds of white blood cells develop in the bone marrow before heading into the bloodstream. Lymphocytes are the white blood cells that deal with bacteria and viruses. Lymphocytes turn into two different kinds of white cells: B cells and T cells.

B cells learn to recognize specific invaders and then produce millions of antibodies that destroy them. Vaccines work by promoting B cells' antibody production. If a live virus or bacteria of the same strain as the vaccine ever enters your body, you will have antibodies ready to fight off the infection. For example, once you've had chicken pox, your body has antibodies ready in case you ever come into contact with that virus again. As a result, you are highly unlikely to have to deal with chicken pox more than once in your lifetime. Other viruses, such as the flu, mutate every year, and as a result we are faced with the possibility of a flu infection almost yearly.

Lymphocytes also evolve into other type of cells called the T cells, or killer T cells. Think of them as special agents that are tasked with finding and eliminating spies. T cells seek out the cells in our body that have already been invaded by viruses and then bump into them to break the membrane and either kill the cell or help it heal. In people with HIV infection, the number of T cells is low and, as a result, their ability to fight off disease is reduced. Even more amazing is the fact that T cells, macrophages and leukocytes communicate. One example of this communication occurs when macrophages find damaged tissue and go to work cleaning it up; they release a chemical called Interleukin-1, which signals and activates T cells to come help heal the injured or infected area.

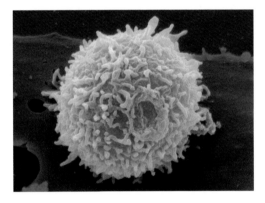

The T cell, one of the immune system's principal means of defence. The T cell will identify the molecular signature of the cell to which it is attached, and if the T cell detects a foe, it will attack.

Every cell in our body that is our own has a marking that allows the immune system to determine if the cell is native or an invader. It's like the IFF (identification, friend or foe) system used by the military. The marker is called the major histocompatibility complex (MCH) or the human leukocyte antigen (HLA). Sometimes the body does not recognize its own cells and thinks that they are invaders. This misidentification occurs in autoimmune diseases such as lupus, celiac disease, type 1 diabetes, inflammatory bowel disease, psoriasis and rheumatoid arthritis, among others. In juvenile onset diabetes, the immune system attacks the cells inside the pancreas that produce insulin. Similarly, in juvenile rheumatoid arthritis, the immune system attacks the tissues inside the joints. Indeed, there are 80 known autoimmune diseases, and they affect almost 7% of the population. Fortunately, new technologies are helping scientists learn more about these diseases, and hope exists for patients with these conditions.

The Lymphatic System

In addition to the bone marrow that produces white cells, the lymphatic system is another critical component of the body's immune system. The lymphatic system filters the blood plasma to trap viruses and bacteria so

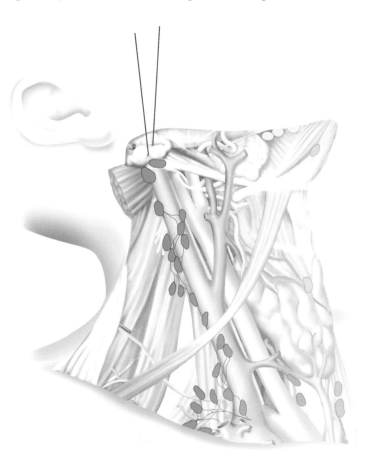

Lymph nodes in the neck (all colours).

they can be disposed of by the cellular components of the immune system. Most people don't know much about the lymphatic system, but when your doctor feels the sides of your neck she is feeling the glands that are part of that system. By checking your lymph glands, your doctor can get an indication whether your body is fighting an infection; when you have one, these glands may swell up and become very sore. The lymphatic system is actually a set of vessels similar to blood vessels that are connected throughout your body. They are filled with a clear fluid called lymph, which is blood plasma—the fluid component of your blood without the red and white blood cells. You've probably seen lymph—when you get a blister, it's usually filled with lymph fluid. Lymph glands, also referred to as lymph nodes, filter fluids from the blood to catch bacteria and viruses or other foreign materials. There are almost 300 nodes in total, with clusters of larger ones in your neck, your underarms and your groin.

The spleen is an organ that lies in your chest cavity. It acts just like the lymphatic system in that it filters the blood, but it also filters out broken or damaged red blood cells in addition to any microbes. It's an interesting organ because it contains concentrated capillary beds that separate the arterial blood (oxygenated blood on its way to the body from the lungs) from the venous blood (deoxygenated blood on its way from the body to the heart). That part of the spleen with loads of capillary beds is called the red pulp. The spleen also has a section called the white pulp, which contains masses of leukocytes and other white blood cells. These cells are highly concentrated and ready to deal with any microbe, damaged or infected cell filtered out of the bloodstream.

TRANSPLANTATION

Even though our immune system and white blood cells are designed to help our bodies and protect us from invasion, sometimes things go wrong. Leukemia is a cancer of the bone marrow that causes huge numbers of abnormal blood cells to be produced and enter the bloodstream. These abnormal white blood cells don't die when they should, causing crowding in the blood that makes it hard, if not impossible, for the other blood cells to do their job.

When I was a post-doctoral fellow at the Hospital for Sick Children, I had the privilege of working with young patients who had leukemia. I did research to see if we could come up with a new method of detecting lung disease in children who had received a bone marrow transplant. Over the three years of the research, I met some remarkable children and their families. Leukemia is treated by aggressive chemotherapy and radiation. The

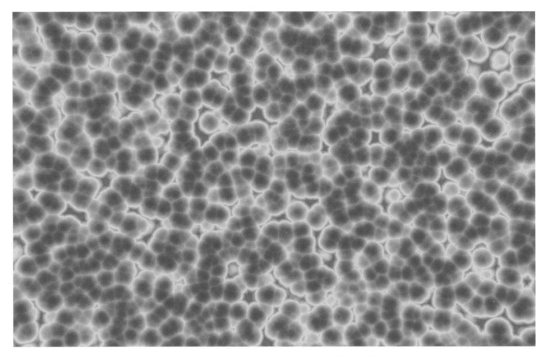

A microscopic image of tissues from the spleen. You can see the red pulp, where the blood is filtered, and the white pulp, where masses of white blood cells are stored. When an invader is sensed in the red pulp, the white cells move in to attack.

treatment is designed to kill off the cancer cells in the bone marrow and blood, with the result that the children become very weak because their red blood cell counts drop to dangerously low levels. Essentially, the doctors take the children as close to death as possible and then bring them back to life in an effort to destroy all the cancer cells in the bone marrow. This treatment is carried out repeatedly to prepare the children for a bone marrow transplant. If they are lucky enough to be matched to a stem-cell donor, then they are eligible for a transplant. Donors have stem cells extracted from their bone marrow, a painful procedure in which a large needle is inserted into the bone. The stem cells are then removed from the donor's bone marrow and injected into the leukemia patient's bone marrow. The stem cells then begin to multiply, creating new bone marrow tissue to replace the old diseased, cancerous tissue. When it works, this treatment is the closest thing to a miracle that I am ever likely to see.

This recognition by the body that it has been invaded, and the resulting all-out assault on the foreign tissue, is the reason why organ transplantation is so difficult. Even though the transplanted tissue, be it heart, lung, kidney or any other organ, is beneficial and needed for survival, the immune system has nevertheless been developed to attack anything that it recognizes as foreign; organ rejection is simply the body's immune system attacking the transplanted organ. Fortunately, great advances have been made in anti-rejection drugs, which control the body's immune system and prevent it from attacking the new organ. Unfortunately, since these drugs dampen the ability of the immune system to fight off all invaders, the organ recipient can become more susceptible to illness in the future. Lung transplant recipients have a very difficult time because the lungs are open to the environment; the air we breathe contains many microbes and viruses that the immune system needs to deal with. Although heart or kidney transplant recipients can reasonably expect to live for many years after receiving their new organs, lung transplant recipients are faced with a much shorter period when they are likely to be free of infection and organ deterioration.

A transplant is amazing to behold, regardless of the potential outcome. During my post-doctoral fellowship at the Hospital for Sick Children, I spent much of my time in the division of respiratory medicine. I was researching the lung disease cystic fibrosis (CF) and I saw some children who were managing the disease well, and others who were having a very hard time. Some children deteriorated significantly and quickly. My colleague Donna Wilkes, the research coordinator for the division, knew most of the children and their families very well, having seen the children every three months for most of their lives. One day she told me that a girl with CF who was on the transplant list had been taken to surgery to receive a lung transplant. Transplantation evokes mixed feelings because you immediately think of the donor who had just passed away and the bravery of their family in donating the organs. It always hits me hard. I've lost friends who donated their organs. A young girl with cystic fibrosis whose lung function had declined so severely that she could barely breathe now had a new lease on life. Donna described the surgery to me—how the patient is placed on life support; how the surgeons saw open the rib cage, take out the diseased

THE KEY VITAMINS FOR HEALTH AND PERFORMANCE

Vitamins A, C, and E. Epidemiological studies show that a high intake of antioxidant-rich foods is inversely related to cancer risk. Antioxidants are recommended after you work out, especially if you have been doing cardiovascular exercise. Foods with lots of antioxidants are likely more effective than supplements. For example, consider adding fresh berries to your smoothie after a workout.

Vitamin A. Carotenoids have been shown to help reduce the risk of breast cancer. Vitamin A has also been reported to improve eyesight. Unfortunately, vitamin A supplementation has also been reported to increase the risk of lung cancer. So if you are a smoker or have a family history of lung cancer, you'd do better eating carrots and foods high in vitamin A than taking supplements.

Vitamin C. Routine administration of vitamin C is recommended in the treatment of hypertension and coronary arterial disease, and following cardiac infarction or stroke. Vitamin C is an antioxidant vitamin and part of the protocol I recommend people consider for post-workout recovery.

Vitamin E. Considerable evidence from basic research, as well as epidemiological evidence, indicates that vitamin E can possbily protect from cardiovascular disease.

Vitamin B12. This vitamin may play a role in the prevention of disorders of the central nervous system development, mood disorders and dementias (including Alzheimer's disease and vascular dementia). This vitamin may have powerful positive effects on the nervous system.

Vitamins B1, B2, B3, B5, B6. A deficient intake of several B vitamins is strongly connected with the development of cancer, neural-tube defects and cardiovascular diseases. Vitamin B complex is also very important in times of higher stress, both mental and physical.

Vitamin D. There may be protective elements in vitamin D that should be part of a cancer-preventive diet, along with selenium and folic acid. It also has positive effects on bone health.

Sources: Borek, 2004; Clarke and Armitage, 2002; Reynolds, 2006; Huang et al., 2006.

infected lungs and then place the new healthy lungs into the patient. What amazed me most about this entire procedure was that this little girl, who had just undergone such a severe procedure, was able to sit up and have a bite to eat eight hours afterward. Her skin colour had gone from grey to a healthy pink for the first time in many months. It is truly an amazing event that captures all the elements of life and death. Given that the first successful transplant, a kidney, happened in 1954, we have made extraordinary progress. We all hope that such progress continues.

THE MIND-BODY CONNECTION

Can you imagine that your brain influences your immune system?

Amazingly, this is true and has major implications for both health and disease. Psychological events that are perceived as negative and stressful by the brain can have a physical effect on the immune system because there are sympathetic nerve connections between the brain and the bone marrow, the thymus, the spleen and the lymph nodes.[48] When electrical signals from the brain descend through these nerves and connect with the various immune system organs, neurotransmitters are released from these nerve endings and circulate through the immune system tissues. The cells of the immune system such as lymphocytes and natural killer cells have receptors on their surface that are sensitive to these neurotransmitters. Therefore, signals from the brain and the nervous system can have a direct impact on the immune system cells, increasing or decreasing their activity levels.

In addition to direct nerve connections between the brain and the immune system, there are also chemical signal connections. Endocrine system organs such as the hypothalamus and the pituitary glands in the brain, or the adrenal glands above the kidneys, release chemical-signalling hormones, including epinephrine (also known as adrenaline), norepinephrine and cortisol, which circulate throughout the body. These hormones produce wide-ranging effects on most body tissues and also affect the white blood cells of the immune system. Just as immune system cells have receptors for neurotransmitters, they also have receptors for hormones. When the hormones bind to the surface of the white blood cells, they have wide-ranging effects on the distribution and function of the cells.

People typically think that the mind and body are separate. Our thoughts don't affect our bodies—how could they? They are just thoughts and don't really even physically exist, right? Actually, this is wrong. Thoughts exist as electrical currents passing through the neurons of our brains. Sometimes those electrical currents pass through areas of the brain that are part of the endocrine system. (For more information, see Chapter 5 on the endocrine system.) When these passages happen, hormones leave the endocrine organs to circulate through the body. We perceive this response as emotions or physical feelings. Imagine you are lying in bed, thinking about something that happened at work. You tense up, your heart rate increases and your breathing rate goes up. These changes are the mind–body stress response. I'll talk about this response in detail in Chapter 7 and provide tips on how to combat the negative effects that go along with it, but it is an important concept to deal with here because psychological stress causes a decrease in the effectiveness of your immune system.

Think back to your high school or university exams. I was one of many people who crammed for finals; perhaps you did so as well. I remember the sleepless nights, the anxiety, the constant memorization, the focusing for hours on end, and the mental fatigue—not to mention overdosing on caffeine and poor food. I also remember getting sick right after exams ended. I got sick on other occasions as well, usually right after stressful life events. Many of the athletes I've coached over the years ended up getting sick right after we finished a training camp or competition. From a societal perspective, we see increasing pressure and stress in the workplace and observe correlations between stress levels and the incidence of sick days claimed by employees. Interestingly, the link between these stressful mental or psychological events and the incidence of illness has a physiological foundation—mental stresses actually affect the immune system and weaken it. Many healthy people are able to resist disease despite temporary stress-induced immunosuppression, but this resistance decreases as we age, or if we have a disease or if the stress levels remain elevated over time. Athletes are therefore at risk because they're under a constant training load that stresses the adaptive abilities of the body; any extra psychological stress has a greater impact on their immune system and health than it might for someone who is not training intensely.

Scientists who serve on expeditions to remote locations such as Antarctica are exposed to extreme isolation for extended periods. The often-dangerous travel to these locations, along with the anxiety of being cut off from friends and family for months at a time, is highly stressful. This psychological stress has a clear impact on the immune system; in fact, measurements of immunoglobulin A and M during an Antarctic expedition made by Dr. Maree Gleeson, from the Hunter Immunology Unit, Royal Newcastle Hospital in the United Kingdom, showed that these markers of specific immunity decreased for the first four months of the expedition and then eventually returned to normal levels.[49] Dr. Gleeson speculated that

GREG'S HIGH-PERFORMANCE TIPS

CAFFEINE COMPROMISES YOUR IMMUNE SYSTEM—AVOID IT WHEN YOU'RE SICK.

Caffeine appears to suppress the immune system as well as the inflammatory response. The anti-inflammatory effect may be helpful in some circumstances, especially with inflammatory diseases, but immune suppression is a major concern. Caffeine does improve mental and physical performance, so it can sometimes help you on an exam or at a key work moment (such as a presentation), if taken only 30 to 60 minutes beforehand. This advice applies to athletes just before competing as well. But chronic constant use—especially at doses higher than the equivalent of two cups per day—can cause problems.

Source: Horrigan et al., 2006.

the decreased immunity may have been caused by the psychological stress of isolation or also by the fact that it takes several months to adapt to the Antarctic cold. NASA and Russian scientists are also conducting research like this in preparation for the planned expedition to Mars, where astronauts will be isolated for many months on the trip to and from the planet.

Dr. Susan Segerstrom from the University of Kentucky and and Dr. Gregory Miller from the University of British Columbia compiled the results from more than 300 empirical studies on the relationship between psychological stress and the immune system.[50] The authors used a technique called a meta-analysis, where the data from each study are combined and then analyzed. In total, their analysis included data from more than 18,000 subjects. They found that responses to acute stress and chronic stress differed. They defined acute stress as events such as public speaking or doing mental arithmetic for between five and 100 minutes. (One of the studies even included parachuting.) These brief, acute stress moments seemed to up-regulate "natural immunity"—the activities of macrophages and natural killer cells that broadly target any kind of invader. For example, after public speaking (an activity most people find terrifying) there are more neutrophils in the bloodstream, as well as cytokines that increase the inflammatory response (interleukin-6), as well as a cytokine that stimulates the activity of macrophages and natural killer cells (interferon gamma—IFN-y). Conversely, short bouts of stress decrease "specific immunity"—immune cells such as antigens that are designed to target specific bacteria or viruses that have built up as part of a learned immune response to a previous infection or immunization. In general, the authors' analysis shows that, in response to a stressful situation, the immune system increases natural immunity that targets many microbial invaders, and decreases specific immunity that has developed to target specific diseases. Simply put, the body is preparing itself to defend against an immediate threat such as an injury, not a long-term problem such as an illness.

This change of emphasis makes sense from an evolutionary perspective because the stress response has developed to deal with environmental threats that, in the past, were likely to cause physical damage. Therefore, to best protect against injuries such as cuts and scrapes, there's an increase in the broad-spectrum immune response to deal with the immediate threat of the open cut, and a shutdown of the response of the acquired immunity cells used to fight bacteria and viruses that we have been exposed to in the past. But viruses and bacteria are evolving as well to overcome the various layers of our immune systems. Some viruses fool the body into shifting toward a natural immune response and away from a specific response. The herpes virus is particularly good at deceiving the body into activating the wrong type of defence mechanism and down-regulating the specific response that the body may have ready for it. The immune system's war against bacteria, viruses and microbes is really like an arms race. The problem with stressors is that they cause the body to shift its limited energy reserves in support of immediate demands. This shift creates openings for invaders to get through our defences, which may cause illness and disease.

Unfortunately, although acute short-term stressors (public speaking, skydiving or exams, for example) can cause a shift in the immune system's focus from one area to another, chronic stress causes a total down-regulation of all aspects of the immune system. Chronic stressors included in Dr. Segerstrom's and Dr. Miller's analysis were events such as caring for a loved one with dementia, dealing with unemployment or adapting to living with an injury or chronic illness. In these cases, all aspects of the immune system were compromised. Chronic stress is known to cause the release of a hormone called cortisol. This hormone has broad effects across the body, but in the context of the immune system, cortisol acts to decrease the function of the various cells of the immune system. For example, the toxicity of natural killer cells is decreased when cortisol levels in the blood are elevated. Tragically, people experiencing chronic stressors such as bereavement or employment loss are often at much greater risk of becoming sick than those not experiencing these life events. Of course, the added burden of personal illness makes getting through a challenging life event much more difficult.

GREG'S HIGH-PERFORMANCE TIPS

SHOULD I EXERCISE WHEN I AM SICK?

People are often uncertain whether to rest or exercise when sick. Most sports medicine experts recommend that if you have symptoms related to the common cold (i.e., above the neck) and do not have a fever, moderate exercise is probably safe. Intense exercise should be avoided because it may suppress the immune system further. If you have symptoms related to the flu, such as fever, extreme fatigue, muscle ache or swollen lymph glands, then you should rest and avoid moderate to intense exercise.

THE IMMUNE SYSTEM AND CHRONIC DISEASE

One of the more interesting discoveries in recent years is that the immune system is involved with the control of cancer. Cancer has proven to be a terribly difficult disease to treat, probably because to some extent "cancer" is a word used to broadly describe many very different diseases that share similar characteristics. But lung cancer is actually a very different disease from pancreatic cancer, prostate cancer and so on. The immune system and the various cells that make up the system's response to infection also serve to combat cancer in the human body. Immune system cells can target and destroy tumour cells or other types of cancer cells, especially certain kinds of lymphomas. However, suppression of the immune system owing to stress or other factors can increase the incidence of cancer. After World War II, researchers monitored the incidence of cancer in a group of 6284 Jewish Israelis who had lost an adult son during the Second World War. There were higher rates of cancer in the bereaved parents than in non-bereaved members of the population. In this case, it appears that the chronic stress response suppressed the immune system and created an opportunity for cancer cells to grow and propagate.

The link between the brain and cancer works in the other direction: Positive psychology has a demonstrable effect on disease outcome. A number of recent studies have clearly demonstrated that psychological interventions, including support groups, relaxation therapy and stress management techniques, improve immune system parameters and survival and decrease metastasis rates (whether or not the cancer spreads to other organs).[51] This causal link among positive psychology, the immune system and cancer outcome has yet to be clarified, but these studies suggest that psychological interventions may be positive additions to the current battery of medical treatments currently available.

In addition to the benefits of positive psychology, the benefits of moderate exercise may actually help prevent and treat cancer.[52] Perhaps the most exciting data come from a number of research studies on mice, rats, guinea pigs and humans showing that moderate exercise increases macrophage function and specifically improves the macrophages' ability to target and destroy tumour cells. Studies have shown benefits in cases of prostate cancer, lung cancer, intestinal tumours, colon lymphoma and other cancers. At the moment, the benefits appear to be most pronounced in prevention of the various cancers, but there may also be benefits in the early stages of such diseases.

The most recent data suggest that regular exercise (30 minutes a day for 5 days a week) decreases cancer risk by 24–50%.[53] Even more revealing is that the volume and intensity of the regular exercise is inversely related to cancer risk, meaning that the more exercise people do, the lower the risk of cancer. This research is relatively new, and more studies are needed to determine the frequency, intensity and duration of exercise required to best prevent and treat

WHAT KIND OF EXERCISE IS BEST IF I HAVE CANCER?

Whenever possible, people with chronic diseases are now recommended to do some light to moderate physical activity and exercise to maintain or even increase their strength, endurance and, ultimately, health. Always check with your doctor to see if exercise will help you. Not everyone should exercise, and there are times when exercise is good for you and times when it should be avoided. For example, it is best not to exercise for about 48 hours after chemotherapy. If your doctor has given you the okay to exercise, always begin very slowly and progress gently. There are many different kinds of cancer, and research on the benefits of exercise for cancer patients is new. So take your time to find the exercise that makes you feel better and that you can incorporate into your life. Simple walking can do wonders for your fitness and energy levels. Other options include swimming, cycling and jogging to build up cardiovascular health and endurance; strength-building exercises such as weightlifting; or flexibility-increasing exercises, including yoga.

different types of cancers. For now, most evidence suggests that moderate exercise has wide-ranging benefits. For more information on how to design exercise training plans, check out the information in Chapters 1, 2 and 7.

Fortunately, there are ways to enhance the immune system and increase its resistance. Many people turn to drugs to try to combat disease, and in some cases this is important and necessary. But there are other, non-pharmaceutical options. Amazingly, some foods improve the function of our immune system, and we have learned from athletes that exercise can improve the immune system as well.

Staying healthy is critically important for athletes at any level, even the recreational athlete. Many of us who are training for health or for fun lose days of training to sickness. And the older we get, the longer it takes to get back to where we were previously. Of course, when you're not feeling well, your family life suffers, along with your ability to perform at your job. Fortunately, by considering all the information in this chapter and following my simple recommendations for avoiding illness, you can maximize your chances of preventing chronic diseases and living a healthy, happy life. Everyone can take simple steps to strengthen their immune system and prevent infection.

Here are the recommendations that I suggest for the athletes I work with:

▶   Exercise at least 30 minutes a day, especially on high-stress days.
▶   Ensure that you eat a balanced diet with plenty of fruits and vegetables.

- ▶ Consider interventions with vitamins and minerals around periods of travel or high stress.
- ▶ Emphasize personal hygiene like washing your hands, especially when you're in high-traffic public places. Avoid touching your eyes, nose or mouth until after you have washed your hands.
- ▶ Rest and sleep as much as feasible during or immediately following stressful periods or travel.
- ▶ Monitor your stress and fatigue levels. Recover and regenerate during and after higher-stress times or travel, or after periods of intense exercise.
- ▶ Avoid exposure to infected individuals.
- ▶ Review vaccinations before travelling.
- ▶ Consult your physician for a physical review at least annually.

Remember, the most important time to guard against illness and infection is during the short period following intense workouts or in times of increased stress.

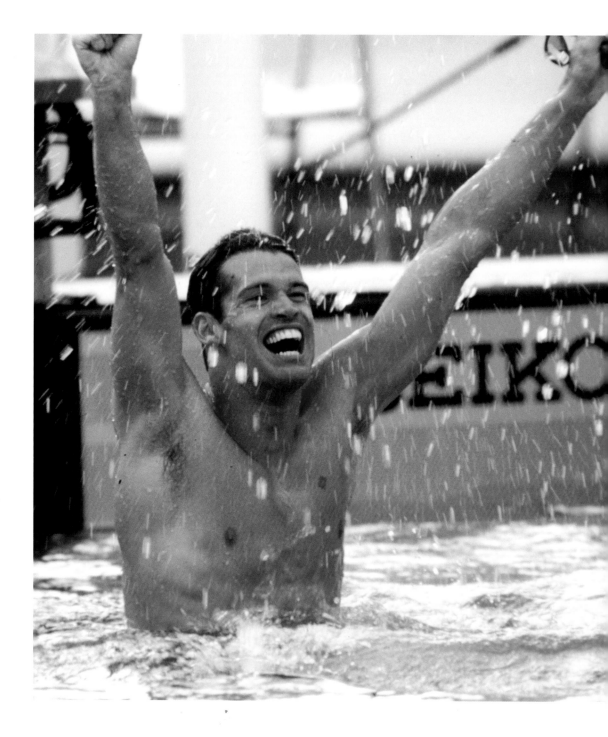

PERFORMING UNDER PRESSURE

THE ENDOCRINE SYSTEM

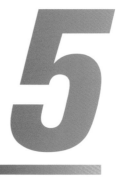

Most of the time when someone says "hormones," we think of the raging hormones in teenagers we know (including our children), or perhaps we remember our own adolescent years. We blame these hormones for teenagers' erratic behaviour, and we know that the changes in the human body during this time are caused by adjustments in hormone levels through adolescence. Although most people are aware that hormones have an impact on teenagers, we are less aware of the powerful impact they have on everyone all the time.

The endocrine system uses hormones to communicate. It is similar to the nervous system, which uses electrical signals to communicate between the various organs, only it works more slowly. Electrical signals are transmitted very quickly, but hormones take some time to be released into the bloodstream and circulate to the target organ. The result is a slower rate of communication, but what the endocrine system loses in terms of speed, it makes up for in the magnitude of the physiological responses it can produce. Think about the last time you were startled, and how several seconds later your heart started pounding in your chest. That's the endocrine system kicking in to activate your body.

More specifically, hormones are special chemicals produced by endocrine glands. There are many of these glands in the human body, each releasing different kinds of hormones. The various hormones have different chemical structures and shapes, allowing them to have specific effects on specific target organs. These target organs have receptors on their surface that are mirror images of the hormone structure, so the hormones can link

129

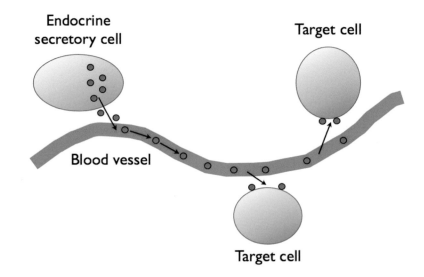

Endocrine
secretory cell

Target cell

Blood vessel

Target cell

Endocrine glands release hormones into the bloodstream, where they travel to target organs.

up with the receptor and precipitate a series of chemical reactions in the target cell. An analogy would be the special connector on the space shuttle that matches a port on the International Space Station. When the space shuttle and the space station link up, information and supplies are transferred and actions occur on the space station as a result. In this chapter, I'll show you some of the key functions of the endocrine system. Let's start with a topic that we're all familiar with—adrenaline.

ADRENALINE AND PERFORMANCE PRESSURE

Hormones have an impact on our physiology and psychology. Indeed, the emotions we experience are mostly the result of circulating hormones. For example, when we are scared suddenly, our bodies respond by releasing adrenaline (also known as epinephrine) into the bloodstream from the adrenal glands above the kidneys. This adrenaline circulates and when it reaches the heart, causes it to start pounding. I had a chance to see and feel the effects of adrenaline up close when I worked at the Barcelona Olympics in 1992.

Watching my friends compete at the Olympics was great, mainly because I got to experience the Olympics without all the pressure. (Okay, I would have given my . . . well, a lot, to be there competing. But it wasn't in the cards.) This was my first experience of the Games, and I worked with a TV crew helping behind the scenes by carrying cables or whatever else they needed. In that Olympics, Mark Tewksbury won a gold medal for Canada in swimming. Mark and I had been teammates in Calgary, so I managed to get assigned to the pool that night to watch the swim. All 20,000 people in the swim stadium were supercharged, because the Spanish hero Martin López-Zubero was swimming in the race just a few days after winning gold in the 200-metre backstroke. The stadium atmosphere was electric. The Brazilian fans were playing music on drums, the Spanish fans were chanting for López-Zubero and most people were singing along. The stands were rocking—literally. (I was on a TV tower that was moving back and forth.) My job was to help film Mark's parents in the stands. It wasn't easy to keep them in the camera shot.

Before swim races the athletes gather in the "ready room," a small room where they stand or sit together before going out to the stadium. They have to stay there for 10 or 15 minutes before each event. Of course, the mind games played there are legendary. But on this occasion, the pressure in the ready room was even greater because the room was directly below the stands where all the Spanish fans were going crazy. I've heard Mark describe the scene, and he tells a great story of just how wild the environment was as he and the other competitors walked onto the deck. Now that I have accumulated much more learning and research, I have an even greater appreciation for that moment. The physiological impact on the human body is tremendous.

The athletes' eyes, ears and skin all pick up the sights, sounds and actual vibrations from the surrounding world. In that supercharged environment, the stimulus is electrifying. Sense organs (eyes, ears, nose, mouth and skin) are connected by nerves to the brain. The brain processes the information it gathers from the environment and decides if there's a threat. Although no life-threatening event was occurring, the presence of TV cameras, the knowledge that a lifetime of work was on the line, and the awareness that 20,000 screaming people were watching would have been translated by the brain as an abnormal situation. It had better get the body ready for action.

Under stress and pressure, the brain activates a critical endocrine system area of the brain—the hypothalamus. It's a small region made up of nerves, secretory cells and blood vessels, and is responsible for the regulation of hunger, thirst, body temperature, water balance and blood pressure. The hypothalamus is connected at its lower part to the command centre of the endocrine system—the pituitary gland. When the hypothalamus is stimulated, it releases a hormone called corticotropin-releasing hormone (CRH), which acts on the pituitary gland, causing it to release adrenocorticotropic

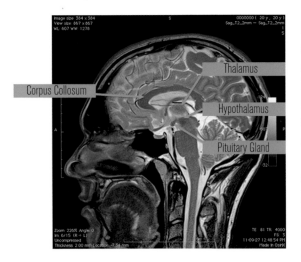

Image size: 384 x 384
View size: 867 x 867
WL: 607 WW: 1278

0000000 (20 y , 20 y)
Sag_T2_2mm — Sag_T2_2mm

Corpus Collosum

Thalamus

Hypothalamus

Pituitary Gland

Zoom: 226% Angle: 0
Im: 6/15 (R + L)
Uncompressed
Thickness: 2.00 mm Location: -7.54 mm

TE 81 TR 4000
F9 5
11-09-27 12:48:54 PM
Made In OsiriX

A cross-section of the brain showing the structures that are associated with the endocrine system.

hormone (ACTH). ACTH enters the bloodstream and travels to the adrenal cortex, which sits at the top of the adrenal glands (above the kidneys). So Mark's adrenal glands, responding to the ACTH from the endocrine glands in the brain, started to secrete epinephrine and cortisol into the bloodstream.

The effects of epinephrine (also known as adrenaline) on the human body are powerful. Most Olympic athletes experience epinephrine. The rest of us have also felt its effects. A startling event or public speaking can cause us to become nervous. The hypothalamic-pituitary-adrenal axis (HPA axis) is activated, causing the release of epinephrine. Epinephrine increases muscle power, the heart beats more quickly and powerfully, the airways in the lungs expand, the eyes dilate to let more light in, and digestive system activity slows as more blood is diverted to the muscles. (This is why our mouths go dry when we are nervous; we have no need for saliva to help digestion when the brain perceives that we're in danger.)

The release of epinephrine into our circulatory system is a response that supercharges the body to prepare it for physical exercise. For Mark Tewksbury at the Barcelona Olympics this was a good thing because he managed to keep his nerves under control and swim to a gold medal. Mark practised mental rehearsal and imagery for months leading up to the Games. This helped him manage his psychological responses to the stressful environment. By the time he walked out to the pool, he had seen the crowd many times before—in his mind. Mental visualization is a powerful stress management skill that anyone can use to help improve performance and health. You can imagine relaxing scenes to help calm your mind and body, or picture successful outcomes to your goals to help improve your motivation—the possibilities are endless. I've listed some basic steps on the left, and if you are interested you can check out some training audio segments by sport psychologist Dr. Peter Jensen.

The interesting theme for me as a scientist engaged in helping athletes prepare for international competitions is that all these successful performers used different mental skills to achieve the same thing: being able to focus only on their performance. This may seem simple, but under the

WHAT HAPPENS WHEN . . . THE HYPOTHALAMUS DOES NOT WORK?

At the Hospital for Sick Children, I had the opportunity to work with a group of patients who had tumours in their hypothalami. These tumours, called craniopharyngiomas, were removed by surgery. Unfortunately, removing the tumours also removes part or all of the hypothalamus. After surgery, the young patients had a very hard time regulating their metabolisms. For example, their sensation of hunger was not related to how much or how little they ate. Similarly, one of the patients felt thirsty constantly. It's unfortunate that patients who have had this surgery often develop obesity because of the dysfunction of the metabolic regulation. I was part of a research team investigating the effectiveness of AMP-kinase, an enzyme that may help patients' mitochondria function more effectively, and therefore improve their metabolisms and responsiveness to exercise. Our initial results have been positive, and we are studying this area further in hopes of developing a proven intervention to help these children.

STRESS AND PERFORMANCE UNDER PRESSURE

I've spent many years as a scientist and exercise physiologist working with Olympic-level athletes. My job has been to look very closely at each Olympic success, dissect it, and examine the difference between the winning performances and the less successful ones. Several key events and moments during the Games in Vancouver had a big impact on me, not only because of the inspiration of the performances, but also because of the way the athletes were able to execute those performances under pressure. Optimum performance under pressure and stress is what success and leadership, in every aspect of life, are all about.

A key moment that captivated me at the Vancouver Olympics was Alexandre Bilodeau's gold-medal performance in moguls. He was the first Canadian to capture gold on home soil, and the shots of Alexandre and his family after the win were moments that will never be forgotten by the Canadians who were watching. But what I noticed most was the 20 seconds before he even started his run. If you ever get a chance to see a replay, watch what Alexandre was doing before the event started. He was nodding his head and repeating a statement to himself as he stood looking down the ski hill. Once he had the ideas that he wanted in his brain (two words: "forward" and "soft"), he began his run. This technique is called positive self-talk. An athlete will repeat a single word or concept to focus the mind before or during a performance. This was very important for Alexandre because the potential for distraction at that moment was significant. We can all apply this technique at critical moments in our lives: before a key presentation, perhaps, or an exam or a music performance. Think about what you need to do to have a great performance and then see if you can describe those actions in one or two words. Then say those words to yourself right before the performance begins to remind yourself of what you need to do to be successful.

USE CUE WORDS TO HELP YOU FOCUS ON CRITICAL ELEMENTS OF YOUR PERFORMANCE

Cue words are statements that serve to remind you about what you should be doing in a challenging situation or what your response to pressure should be. The heat of the moment often causes us to react without thinking or acting properly. Cue words can help you to think before you respond. The following steps will help you establish your own cue words.

1   List challenging situations and some key skills that will help you achieve your goals.
2   Describe an ideal way to respond to these situations.
3   Try to find one word or phrase that summarizes the response that you should have.

When you're under a deadline or facing pressure, use your cue word to remind you to act as you have planned.

magnifying glass of the Vancouver Olympic Games, it was not an easy thing to achieve. The Olympics are inspiring because we see athletes with whom we can identify as they perform or struggle under pressure. We all face equivalent challenges to perform or struggle (although the pressure is different). Stress and pressure have a profound impact on our bodies and activate our endocrine system.

CHANGES IN HORMONES WITH REST

Some hormones, such as testosterone, have an anabolic effect in that they help build and repair tissue. Others, such as cortisol, have a catabolic effect—they facilitate instant performance improvements, but stop adaptation. Scientists have studied the relationship between anabolic and catabolic hormones and how the levels of these hormones change before and during sport competition. They have noted a significant correlation between the increase of the testosterone (anabolic):cortisol (catabolic) ratio and improvement in performance during a four-week taper.[54] Changing the balance between anabolic and catabolic hormones may improve recovery after exercise and speed the elimination of fatigue. This finding suggests a particularly important consideration for athletes and coaches—the elimination of extraneous stress during taper.

This type of stress reduction is particularly important for people in leadership positions. Simply put, chronic stress changes hormone levels in the body in such a way that positive adaptations, recovery and regeneration are impaired. Most people experience some fatigue and stress over the course of a day and throughout the workweek. To recover properly, our physiological stress levels have to be decreased so that anabolic hormones can take over. When we are in a position of leadership (e.g., as a coach, a teacher or another mentor) or in a supervisory position at work, we have a powerful effect on the stress levels of the people with whom we work. This effect can be either positive or negative. A lot depends on what we all need to accomplish. Obviously, we can push people to a higher stress level in the short term if we need to achieve something quickly. But this may not always be desirable.

Reducing any type of stress, even the kind not related to sports (e.g., travel, exams or presentations), can reduce the level of cortisol and improve positive adaptation. In sports, this finding implies that the added stress from higher-than-normal levels of anxiety and nervousness that occur as major competitions approach must be accounted for in the taper protocol. Coaches can reduce competition anxiety and travel stress by easing training levels or through sport psychology techniques such as visualization and progressive relaxation. For the

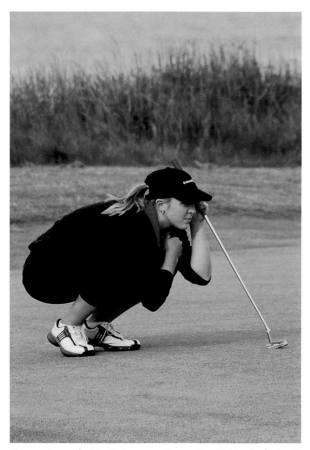

Elite amateur golfer Kira Meixner practices putting. Sinking the final putt to win a tournament can be extremely stressful. Golfers need to control their bodies, their minds and their emotions in order to be able to execute precise shots under pressure.

rest of us—those who aren't athletes but are still interested in improving our own performance at critical times—the lesson is that reducing negative stress in the days leading up to the event is crucial. This works when we prepare for a key presentation, writing exams or performing onstage.

Take Joannie Rochette's performance at the 2010 Winter Olympics. Joannie's mother had passed away suddenly only days before. Joannie went on to the ice and became emotional at the beginning of her performance. She then returned to speak to her coach who, to her credit, was entirely positive and energetic. You could see this in her body language and facial expressions. This was brilliant leadership. Joannie's coach was acting the way Joannie needed to feel: positive, happy, energetic and calming. There was no empathy or physical reflection of nervousness or of the pain and sadness that her coach also must have been feeling. This type of behaviour can lead others to higher levels of performance. The approach should be applied to the taper phase (or to the performance preparation phase) in areas like music, drama, academics or business.

FIGHT OR FLIGHT—THE STRESS RESPONSE

Stress is a somewhat vague term we use for describing our feelings when we are under pressure. Exam stress, family stress, relationship stress, work stress—just reading these words probably sends shivers down your spine. (It is probably sending signals down your HPA axis—that is, the hypothalamus/pituitary gland activation that I described earlier.) In fact, there's a complete range of stresses, and this range has both psychological effects (e.g., increased concentration or anxiety) and physical effects (e.g., increased heart rate or possibly increased heart disease). The short-term effects of acute stress include decreased concentration and increased heart rate. The long-term effects of chronic stress include higher anxiety and heart disease. My point is that stress is critical for increased performance. But if stress is constantly high, then we are at risk of disease. However, by understanding the physiology of stress, we can use it as a performance tool. Our understanding can help us manage the effects of stress so that it does not have an impact on our health. As you will see, I think stress can actually improve our health.

Dr. Hans Selye, a leading stress physiologist, defined stress as the non-specific response of the body to any demand made on it. The psychophysiology of stress is fascinating. Let's use the example of public speaking—which many people fear. We can all relate to being nervous while speaking in front of a room full of people.

When you stand at the front of the room to start your presentation, sensory nerves transmit information to the brain. Specifically, the light entering your eyes causes nerve signals to pass through the optic nerve to the brain. This signal stimulates the limbic system. The limbic system, sometimes called the "emotions brain," organizes and controls many of the complex emotional behaviours and sensations that we experience. Emotions such as pain, pleasure, anger, fear, sadness, attraction and affection all have their roots in the limbic system. The thalamus gland is the first component

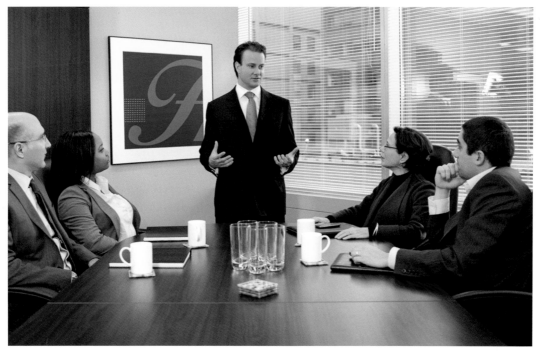

When preparing for a presentation, rehearsal can make a difference. With rehearsal the brain no longer perceives a stressful situation as a threat, so your endocrine system stays calm, your heartbeat remains steady and your palms don't sweat.

of the limbic system activated as a result of nerve impulses from sensory organs during a stress response. This gland, which sits right above the hypothalamus in the middle of the brain, passes messages to the hypothalamus. The hypothalamus in turn activates the various endocrine organs that modulate the stress response. The HPA axis is activated (as described above), and adrenaline/epinephrine is released, along with cortisol, another hormone from the adrenal glands. Cortisol is commonly associated with the stress response.

THE STRESS HORMONE: CORTISOL

Cortisol has widespread effects on metabolism throughout the body. The immediate effects serve to prepare the body for action, because the fight or flight stress response has evolved to protect the body from a perceived threat. So cortisol acts on organs such as the liver to pump glucose into the blood. Glucose is a sugar used as fuel in the brain, and for anaerobic metabolism in the muscles. The immediate effect of cortisol can therefore be felt as an improvement in both brain energy—perhaps an increase in concentration—and muscle energy. Cortisol has powerful anti-inflammatory effects as well. For example, physicians use cortisone (a molecule similar to cortisol) to decrease local inflammation at injury sites. But cortisol also suppresses the immune system, specifically reducing the production of T cells and antibodies. (See Chapter 4 for more information.)

Cortisol is therefore a powerful anti-stress hormone in the short term and can improve mental and physical performance. But problems arise if stress—and, consequently, cortisol levels—remains elevated for long periods. The resulting effects are often the opposite of those produced with short-term cortisol release.[56] They include lipogenesis (fat creation), increased visceral obesity (accumulation of fat tissue in the abdominal cavity around the organs), hyperglycemia (elevated blood sugars), breakdown of tissues and long-term suppression of the immune system. These long-term effects are linked to increased risk of cardiovascular disease, obesity, diabetes and cerebrovascular disease (i.e, stroke).

Nevertheless, our physiological response to stress can be a powerful tool that improves mental and physical performance in the moment—and this result can help us perform at a higher level. The elevated adrenaline and cortisol levels provide our brains with fuel and prime our bodies for physical performance and exercise. These actions can help athletes improve their competitive performance, businesspeople make great presentations, or musicians execute a complicated piece during a performance. But stressors seem to come at us too quickly, and the challenge for all of us is to create times during the day when we can relax and recover. I outline several recovery strategies in Chapter 6. Exercise has been widely proven to reduce not only stress itself, but also most of its physiological effects, such as chronically elevated levels of stress hormones. A simple walk after a presentation or other challenging situation can work wonders. Yoga, Tai Chi and meditation are also excellent options. Remember, 15 minutes of exercise can be enough to change your body's physiology, so take the time each day to recover from stressful events.

Another powerful tool for fighting chronic stress is good food. Eating well provides the foundation for human performance and health and is critical for managing the stress response. Injections of cortisol in human and animal experiments have shown increased appetite, greater cravings for sugar and weight gain.[57] Having found cortisol receptors in the hypothalamus, researchers hypothesize that the greater levels of circulating cortisol may act directly on the hypothalamus to increase the sensations of hunger and cravings for sweets and fats. This link is likely the psychophysiological reason why people eat "comfort foods" in times of stress. Unfortunately, this is the last thing you need then. You can fight the long-term stress response by eating complex carbohydrates (e.g., whole-wheat products, brown rice) rather than foods high in simple sugars. You can also choose good fat options such as avocado, oily fish (e.g., salmon), omega-3 supplements and cold-pressed extra virgin olive oil. You can never go wrong with snacking on organic vegetables and fruit (fruit in moderation). These choices will supply your body with the energy and nutrients it needs to perform—without the negative effects of simple sugars and poor-quality fats.

EUSTRESS—GOOD STRESS AND POSITIVE PRESSURE

Physiologist Dr. Hans Selye also stated that stress can be broken down into distress (bad stress) and "eustress" (good stress). He suggested that the body adapts to each type of stress by altering its internal physiology. It was his belief that these physiological changes were the same regardless of whether the stressor resulted in a eustress or a distress response. The majority of people have negative experiences at both very low and very high levels of stress. The comfortable zone for most people exists somewhere between having nothing to do and being constantly overtaxed by excessive activity. From this idea came the "inverted U" hypothesis.

Athletes are trained to work within a specific performance zone. This zone is often termed the "ideal performance state" (IPS). The IPS is a terrific tool to help you understand the effects of a lack of stress or too much stress on your performance. Looking at the IPS graph on page 142, you can see that it resembles an inverted U—hence the name of the hypothesis. For example, if you have little motivation to complete your work, your performance is likely to be quite poor. At the other end of the spectrum, high activation also results in poor performance. If you are extremely nervous before a public speaking engagement, then the various effects of stress

WHAT CAN I DO TO CONTROL MY STRESS LEVELS?

Your physical responses to stress are the easiest to recognize and reduce quickly and effectively. Use these techniques to increase your resistance to stress.

1   Take three deep, slow breaths and relax. (For comparison, try breathing short, fast, shallow breaths for one minute and see how you feel.) This breathing exercise takes about 15 seconds and works really well if you feel like you're about to blow up.

2   Take a moment and consciously relax your face, shoulders, hands, stomach muscles, back, legs and feet. Let the tension melt away into the floor. Notice how different it feels to be tense as opposed to relaxed. This exercise is especially effective for preventing tense muscles and headaches. Remind yourself to do this tension-release exercise several times a day.

3   Force yourself to smile. Smiling can instantly alter your mood and promote relaxation of muscles. Just contract the muscles in your face that you use to smile and see what happens. Then grimace for a minute, and see if that changes your attitude.

Altering your mental responses to stress is challenging, but with practice the following techniques can help reduce frustration, anxiety and other reactions.

1   Look at the situation and ask yourself if your reaction is really appropriate. Will the event make a difference to you in a week, a month, a year or even five years? This process is called a perspective check. It can help you evaluate your environment in a more positive way and direct your responses more appropriately.

2   Look at your situation and focus on the positive. For example, if you get a promotion, try to see the opportunities for challenges and rewards as well as the increased hours and responsibilities.

on your body will most likely result in an inability to concentrate and other mental and physical effects that make performing on stage almost impossible. But in the middle of the graph lies the ideal performance state. If you want to learn more about the mental skills that help you manage in various performance situations, check out Dr. Peter Jensen's book *The Inside Edge*.

The IPS is the zone where we find an optimal level of excitement, motivation and stress. In this zone, you experience high levels of energy, concentration, enjoyment and accomplishment. We all have an IPS; the challenge is to figure out where it is for you. When I was a competitive swimmer, I had to move into a higher range of activation to be able to perform well. I knew that success depended on being able to move into the upper end of the ideal performance state. I did so by visualizing that I had reached my goals—hyperventilating, jumping explosively and

3   Develop the ability to daydream about a comforting place that you associate with complete relaxation and contentment, such as a favourite vacation spot or a reading chair at home. When you think about such places, you can get your body to respond in a similar way, as if you were really there. You will discover yourself relaxing, breathing slowly and feeling in a better mood. A five-minute mental break can do wonders to help you reset and refocus.

Pay attention to nutrition. The foods we eat are the most important source of energy that we use to think, move and function during the day. The saying "you are what you eat" is very true—much of the body's mass is replaced and repaired by what we eat. Here are a few tips that can improve your resistance to stress:

1   Stay well hydrated. Try to work up to drinking 8 to 10 cups of water each day. Being well hydrated allows your body to store and use energy most effectively.
2   Control your use of caffeine carefully. Caffeine takes half an hour to work and lasts for up to 6 hours, so use it when you need to perform at your best during the day, not all day. Fewer than 2 cups of coffee a day has not been shown to be detrimental to health, but more than 2 cups may increase frustration and anxiety, decrease concentration and cause various health problems.
3   Stay away from salt because it may raise blood pressure (a side effect of stress), and avoid sugars and refined flour because they require vitamin B to be processed. Your body uses vitamin B to fight the effects of stress.

These suggestions require you to break old habits and build new ones. Remember that *perfect* practice makes perfect— set goals and work slowly toward changing your lifestyle to reduce your stress.

generally "psyching up." Interestingly, in my new role as a broadcaster, I've discovered that I need to be in almost the same zone when I'm doing sport science analysis on TV. It's a live performance. I need to be psyched up and energized, and it helps me get focused to concentrate on the task at hand. I think the energy level I try to achieve also helps to convey the passion I have for the topics I'm talking about. But this factor is only one aspect of performance. Sometimes peak performance demands other levels of activation. I find that I have to be very relaxed to learn or to think. I also find that, when I'm in a meeting with colleagues or staff to discuss topics of interest, it's imperative to be not only focused, but also relaxed. Therefore, I've discovered through trial and error (many errors, actually) that I have different performance zones for different tasks. Simple repetitive tasks can be accomplished more quickly by moving my stress to the

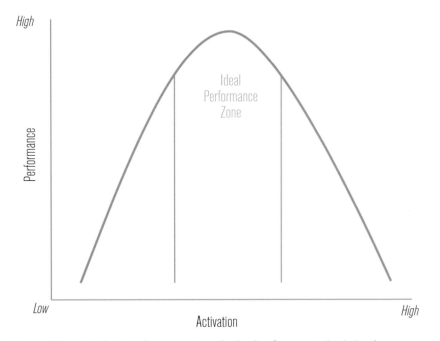

High

Performance

Ideal
Performance
Zone

Low   High

Activation

This graph shows the relationship between activation level and performance. In the ideal performance zone there is a balance between excitement and energy and calm and control.

right along the curve. But more complex tasks, or tasks that require some learning, necessitate staying relaxed. So performing on the left side of the curve can also result in high performance. Each zone needs to be used at the right time.

We all have different zones that are best for our performances. What is your ideal zone for family interactions? At work? In your training? Once you know these zones, you can take steps to move into your IPS whenever it matters. Use the techniques I've presented to help you relax before a key presentation or meeting. Go for a walk to calm down after a moment of high stress during the workday. Psyche yourself up by imagining your success to build motivation and move to the right along the IPS curve.

PSYCHOLOGICAL FACTORS IMPROVE DURING TAPER IN SUCCESSFUL PERFORMERS

Resting has physical benefits, but there are psychological effects as well. Taper time is probably the time of the year that athletes love the most. But it's also the time that coaches like the least because, suddenly, a team of highly disciplined athletes has a ton of energy—all at the same time. When I was coaching, parents would call me the week before a major meet, convinced that something was wrong with their children. Why?

ENTERING YOUR IDEAL-PERFORMANCE STATE (IPS): THE ZONE

Controlling your ideal-performance state (IPS) is a simple, effective way to improve your health, your ability to perform your job and, most importantly, the way you feel. The ideal-performance state is a moment of exceptional achievement—when everything flows, when you are "in the zone." It is usually rare and is often involuntary. However, if you consistently apply the techniques and tips that follow, I believe you'll be able to perform at your best and feel well whenever you wish.

So what *is* your ideal-performance state? Let's begin by thinking about how you were (1) acting, (2) thinking and (3) feeling when performing at your best at a task that was, or is, important to you. Just think about the important things you do that are key to your success. Write down some words that best describe how you act, think and feel when you perform at your best. This is your ideal performance state. Once you know what you were doing, thinking and feeling, it is more likely you'll be able to conjure up those thoughts and emotions again. The next thing to do is to think about a period when you were having a very hard time performing these tasks. How did you act, think and feel? Write down all these.

Research has shown that the typical characteristics of the ideal-performance state include clearly focused concentration and attention, effortless yet intense performance, a lack of analysis, judgment and thought, and feelings of flow. The key to entering your IPS is to act, think and feel in a way that's consistent with your best performance. If you find yourself acting, thinking and feeling in a way that's not in line with what you need to do, take control. Make some changes. Move differently, think differently. Force yourself to be your best under pressure. You can use cue words, tension release or any other tool to make this happen.

Congratulations! You have just completed the first step in learning how to get into your ideal-performance state whenever you really need to. Always try to be aware of what your mind and body are doing as you perform important tasks or responsibilities. Notice and remember the things that help you, and then use them again in the future. If you would like one of our IPS worksheets, just send me a note using the Contact Us page at www.drgregwells.com.

Because they became almost uncontrollable at home, thanks to all the boundless energy. I would explain what was happening and reassure the parents that we would start training hard soon; their kids would be tired and well-behaved in a couple of weeks. From a more scientific perspective, researchers have used a tool called the Profile of Mood States questionnaire to measure tension, depression and anger in athletes during taper. Significant reductions in total mood disturbance and fatigue, as well as other benefits, including increased motivation, arousal and psychological relaxation, were all observed after only one week of a reduced workload. Perhaps this effect is the reason we all feel so great after a week of vacation. We can take advantage of this in our everyday lives because the psychological responses to reduced workloads begin in as little

WORK CYCLING

Our working world is busy and stressful, and this situation is not likely to change. In fact, volatility in our world is the new normal. So we have to find ways to recover and regenerate, just as athletes do when they are training. I recommend that we all take structured and scheduled breaks from our work activities, and I call this routine "work cycling." Work cycling is taking time to recover and regenerate daily (for one hour), monthly (three days of no work/email /etc.) and yearly (two complete weeks off each year). Although these breaks may seem almost impossible to fit in, they are a critical practice that high performers need to adopt to ensure that we have long and productive careers but are still able to maintain our mental and physical health.

as 24 hours. Of course, the success of this factor depends on your ability to relax and not to worry about what you are missing during your personal mini-taper. I use 24-hour mini-tapers when I know I have critical performance moments coming up. When I'm disciplined enough to implement a mini-taper in my own schedule, I inevitably perform at a higher level.

ENDORPHINS AND PAIN

I'm not much of a runner. I love running and it gets me into shape faster than any other form of exercise, but it just does not come easily. As a result, when I read about people who experience the "runner's high," I feel a little envious. I've certainly never felt that way running. I have felt exhilaration on some long bike rides and during some swimming practices. So, to a limited extent, I can identify with this feeling. But in the running world, the runner's high does seem to happen with some regularity. If you've ever experienced it, you may describe it as a feeling of euphoria that occurs when you're working at a very high level. It turns out that this phenomenon can be explained physiologically.

It all comes down to a little hormone called an endorphin. The name endorphin comes from "endogenous" and "morphine," meaning that endorphins are a form of morphine that is created in the human body. More specifically, β-endorphins, which produce a runner's high, are manufactured in the pituitary gland. They are released directly into the bloodstream in response to stress or physical trauma, and they have widespread effects on the nervous system. Receptors for this neuro-hormone are found in the structures that make up the limbic system in the brain. β-endorphins bind to receptors on the surface of nerve cells and act to block sensory signals from the body that are passing to the brain. Therefore, pain signals may be blocked if β-endorphins have been released.

The simple act of exercising causes a release of endorphins into the blood. In 2008, Dr. Henning Boecker used a technique called positron emission tomography (a PET scan) to show that exercise does in fact cause endorphins to be released from the pituitary gland.[58] Participants in this research were highly trained runners who had their brains scanned before and after a two-hour run. Dr. Boecker's results showed that endorphins were produced during exercise. He also showed that the endorphins attach to receptors in parts of the brain that are associated with emotions (the amygdala, the periaqueductal grey matter, the hypothalamus and the medial thalamus), and that the amount of endorphins produced by the runners matched the mood changes they reported. Although there are likely other hormones involved in the sensation of the runner's high, the recent research is a very interesting first step for developing a better understanding of this phenomenon. Unfortunately for me, knowing why people feel a runner's high does not help me keep up with my wife on her training runs.

As I mentioned, β-endorphins are released from the pituitary gland following a stressful or traumatic event. They bind to receptor sites in the nervous system and can, among other things, block incoming sensory signals from the body related to pain. Unlike with the runner's high, I do have some experience with the pain aspect. During another moment of misadventure on my cycling trip through Africa, I had a crash in Malawi. A group of us were cycling on a reasonable road in a pace line—riding in a line, one right after the other as close as possible to the rider in front to reduce wind resistance. You can see a real pace line on page 146 in the picture I took at the 2007 Tour de France. (The eventual winner, Alberto Contador, is in the yellow jersey, and his teammate George Hincapie is right in front of him.)

On that day in Malawi, we were cycling at a reasonable pace. When riding in Africa, you get used to the presence of animals of all shapes and sizes on the roads. Some are worth attention; dogs, for example, like to chase cyclists. But others, like cows, are normally relatively passive. I did not realize that in Malawi there's a cow that also likes to chase—and run into—cyclists as they go by at 35 kilometres an hour. As we were cycling by, a cow charged our group. We swerved to avoid it, and I crashed on some gravelly pavement. Normally, this would not be a big deal. I had some pretty good scrapes down my arms and hip and some damage to a thumb and fingers. (My hand had been caught between the handlebars and the ground when I fell.) In North America, I'd go to the emergency room at the local hospital, get cleaned up and stitched, and then just be sore for a few days during the recovery.

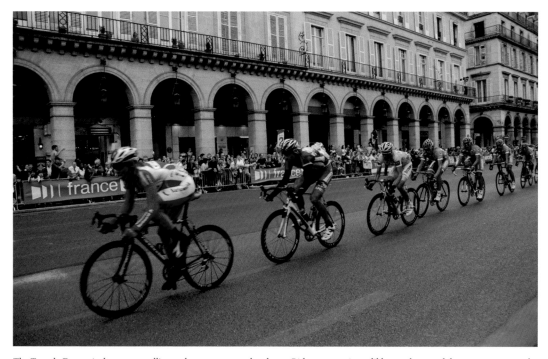

The Tour de France is the most gruelling endurance race on the planet. Riders race at incredible speeds up and down mountains, only inches away from other each other. The endocrine system helps them stay calm, energized and focused.

But in Malawi, I was at least 48 hours from a reasonable hospital. So my friends put some hand sanitizer on my cuts. We got back on our bikes because we had to ride to the next point to reach our support truck, about 40 kilometres away. Interestingly, despite the fact I had hit the ground pretty hard and had many cuts that were bleeding, I really did not feel much pain. Clearly, the trauma of hitting the ground had triggered the release of β-endorphins. They blocked my pain receptors, and I was able to ride to the rest stop and get help from our brilliant nurse (thanks, Kogie).

β-endorphins have a half-life of about 2 hours, which means every 2 hours half of the hormones are broken down. This explains why I started to feel pain only later in the evening. My entire body began to ache, the cuts became extremely sore and it was painful to move. My endorphins were wearing off. The recent discoveries related to endorphin physiology and exercise can also explain some of the stories told of professional soccer or hockey players who continued to play despite having broken bones. The hormones released during exercise and competition simply blocked pain receptors and allowed the players to keep going. This ability is clearly an evolutionary adaptation to allow us to keep moving and performing despite being injured.

My own experiences with pain and endorphins pale in comparison to what polar guide Hannah McKeand described to me during our expedition to the mountains of Bolivia. Hannah has skied from the coast of Antarctica to the South Pole five times, more than anyone else in history. (In her solo and unsupported expedition in 2006, she set a new world speed record for the journey.) Her expeditions usually cover 950 to 1100 km over a 50- to 60-day period in one of the harshest environments on Earth. The ambient temperature usually sits around -20 to -30°C, and the environment can contribute to some of the most unpleasant conditions a human body can endure. Here's how Hannah described her experiences with pain in extreme conditions:

There are two main categories of pain that one will typically encounter on a long polar expedition. The most common is the long-term, slow-developing pain one would experience with a muscle, tendon or ligament that is being subjected to continual repetitive stress over long periods of time. This type of pain can build to almost unbearable levels and at times can mean the end of an expedition without proper attention. The trouble is that there is no adrenaline associated with this kind of pain, it just creeps into you and overwhelms you over a long period. Such pain can of course be tackled with drugs, taping and topical agents, but I have also had a lot of success, both personally and with clients, using visualization and mental strength to deal with long-term pain. I try to imagine the edges of the pain as though the pain is radiating out from the injury like a big invisible sphere. Often the sphere seems enormous, stretching even outside my body. Then I start to focus on making the sphere smaller. I focus on all the parts of my body that aren't in pain, that are functioning normally and without discomfort. As you concentrate, the pain sphere becomes smaller and smaller until it is reduced to something very specific and concentrated in the area of the injury, and your predominant awareness is of the rest of your body that is fine. By exercising this controlled refocusing, I imagine that I am taking control of the pain messaging system my body is trying to communicate a problem with, and forcing it to get some practical perspective. It is like saying, "Calm down! I know my knee is injured! You don't have to keep on about it!

The second type of pain that sometimes occurs is the sudden and unexpected pain that relates to an accident. In 2008, I made an attempt to become the first woman to go solo to the North Pole. Two weeks into the expedition and hundreds of miles from assistance, I had a nasty accident. I had unclipped from my sled and skied up into an area of severely disturbed ice to try and find a route through. There was a lot of blown snow in drifts over the hidden obstacles, and as I was scouting about I suddenly fell through the ice into a deep crack. My injuries were quite extensive. I semi-dislocated an already loose shoulder to the point that I lost movement in the lower arm and feeling in several of my fingers. I cracked two ribs, twisted and nastily pulled my left hip flexor, severely aggravated a herniated disk in my lower back and bruised myself black and blue. Strangely, as I landed in a tangled and mangled mess in the bottom of my hole, I scrambled to my knees and the only injury I was initially aware of was my bitten tongue which was bleeding profusely onto the ice in front of me. The adrenaline and endorphins were pumping through me with such intensity immediately after the fall that it was several minutes before I began to be aware that I was actually quite badly hurt. I was trapped in the hole for over an hour while I puzzled out how to use a ski as a makeshift ladder that would send me slithering out of my prison on my belly, and for most of that frightening and stressful period I was only dimly aware of the pain I was in. There were sharp, aggressive stabs of pain related directly to aggravating my injuries trying to climb out, but mostly I was just focused on escape. The moment I succeeded and managed to drag myself into my tent I quickly began to feel like I'd been run over by a train. And the next day I could hardly move at all.

Fortunately, Hannah was able to extricate herself from the hole and set up a camp, where she waited several days until she was rescued by a Russian helicopter.

MELATONIN, THE PINEAL GLAND AND SLEEP

As I've explained, hormones have powerful effects on the human body. But did you know they are responsible for that drowsy feeling you get in the evening? A hormone called melatonin is closely involved in the sleep process. It is secreted from the pineal gland, a tiny organ in the middle of your brain right behind the eyes. The production of melatonin

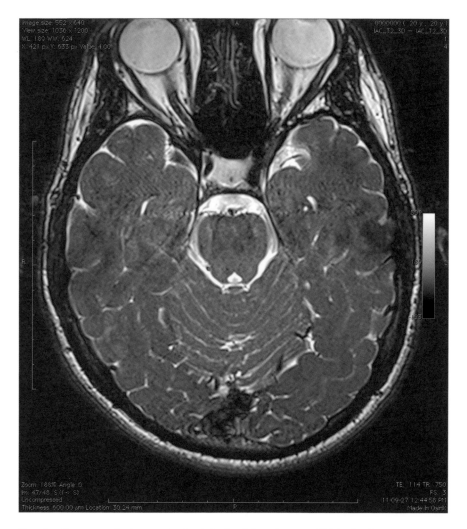

There is a direct connection between the pineal gland and the optic nerve, which is why it's important to sleep in a dark room in order to achieve good-quality sleep.

is increased 50-fold at night. Levels of melatonin released from the brain increase during the course of the evening, peak during the night and then decrease during the day. Production during the day is decreased because the pineal gland is sensitive to bright light. There are direct nerve connections from the optic nerve to the pineal gland. This is why it is so important to keep your room dark at night, and why, if possible, you should avoid turning on lights during the night—for instance, when you're going to the bathroom at 2 a.m. The light stimulus can turn off

IMPROVEMENTS IN SLEEP WHEN ATHLETES REST BEFORE COMPETITION

A study on female swimmers demonstrated an improvement in sleep duration and perceived quality during taper.[59] An improvement in sleep quality is important because growth hormone is released during stages 3 and 4 sleep, and naturally released growth hormone acts to repair muscle tissue and speed recovery. There are a number of physiological changes in the body that happen at different times when we sleep, and these are referred to as "sleep stages." I recommend getting at least eight hours of sleep during a taper phase before competition or the night before any important performance event. New research also suggests that you should take advantage of an afternoon nap to bump the total amount of sleep even higher and improve your mental performance in the afternoon.

melatonin production and disrupt the quality of your sleep. In the evening, increased melatonin levels cause the blood vessels in the skin to dilate, releasing body heat into the environment and cooling the body by 0.3–0.4°C. This cooling promotes drowsiness and helps us fall asleep. As an aside, if you have travelled across time zones and are having a hard time falling asleep, have a cool shower to decrease your body temperature slightly, and then make sure your room is as dark as possible. This procedure mimics the effect of melatonin and can help you fall asleep in the new time zone.

Melatonin release is cyclic and not totally dependent on light. The cyclic nature of pineal gland activity is the reason we get jet lag. The circadian rhythm, generated by structures in the brain, provides some direct input to the pineal gland, telling it when to release melatonin on a roughly 25-hour cycle. When we travel to a new time zone, the pineal gland is activated on the old schedule. This pineal gland activity can cause you to feel very drowsy in the middle of the day, and wide awake in the middle of the night—problematic for business travellers or athletes who have to perform during the day in the new time zone.

I have worked with the Canadian amateur golf team for many years. On several occasions, head coach Dean Spriddle and I took a group of athletes to compete in the British amateur tournament. Our challenge was to help the athletes play at an elite international level less than 36 hours after leaving North America for the United Kingdom. We developed a strategy to minimize the effects of jet lag and speed adaptation to the new time zone. Golf is a precision sport, so helping the athletes adapt was crucial. Jet lag has been shown to impair motor performance and mental performance, as well as producing a general sensation of fatigue.

Fortunately, by exposing our eyes to light first thing in the morning, we were able to speed the resetting of our body clocks. Regardless of how

MANAGING JET LAG

If you are travelling east (e.g., from North America to Europe), you will be predisposed to better performance in the early afternoon on the first few days after arrival. For best results, schedule meetings or sport events for that time.

Of course, the opposite is true if travelling west. To give yourself the best chance of performing on demand, schedule important tasks for the morning on the first few days of arrival. Here are some other tips for the traveller:

▶ Drink 1 litre of water for every three hours in the air during flights to avoid dehydration. My simple rules are 1 litre within North America, 2 litres between North America and Europe or South America, and 3 litres between North America and the Middle East or Asia.

▶ Avoid caffeine while flying.

▶ Exercise in the morning on arrival in the new time zone.

▶ The day before you travel, eat snacks and small meals throughout the day rather than larger meals at breakfast, lunch and dinner.

▶ The day you arrive, eat normal meals at the new time zone schedule. This practice will help reset your body clock.

▶ Expose yourself to natural light as much as possible in the new time zone, and keep your room very dark in the evening and at night.

tired we were after the overnight flight, we got off the plane and immediately went outside into the light and fresh air. We ate breakfast at the local breakfast time. We didn't take naps during the day—even in the early afternoon, when our bodies were used to falling asleep (it was five hours later, according to our internal body clocks). The next morning, we woke up early and went outside into the light. We also exercised for about 30 minutes to increase our core body temperatures. This exposure to light and morning exercise helped shut off melatonin release and moved our clocks ahead very quickly.

Another trick we used was to make our hotel rooms totally dark at about 8 p.m., local time. Even though it was still light outside, walking into a dark room with not even the TV on shut off any inhibition from the optic nerve to the pineal gland, allowing melatonin release to begin earlier than normal. We coupled this early darkness with very hot then cool showers to decrease body temperature and help prepare for sleep. These practices— exposing yourself to light or dark, exercising in the morning in the new time zone, and controlling your body temperature in the evening—can help you perform in business or sports, and even enjoy your vacation more if you're travelling east or west.

Unfortunately, melatonin levels decrease as we age, starting at about age 40. This decrease may be why older people have trouble sleeping. New research suggests that a melatonin supplement may be recommended for people over 40. Check with a naturopathic doctor in your area if you think this may be an option to explore.

GROWTH HORMONE

If you Google "human growth hormone" (HGH), you will generate hundreds of thousands of results, many of them sites that sell synthetic HGH or some older product purporting to reverse the aging process. Human growth hormone is released from the pituitary gland in response to stress, malnutrition and exercise. Secretion of HGH varies throughout the day, with the greatest concentrations during stages 3 and 4 of sleep. The highest level of HGH occurs in our teenage years and then declines slowly thereafter; hence, the marketing of this hormone as the fountain of youth.

Growth hormone exerts its effects by binding to a specific receptor on the surface of target organs. These receptors are found in the liver, heart, kidneys, intestine, lungs, pancreas, cartilage, adipose tissue (fat) and skeletal muscle. Among other effects, HGH stimulates calcium retention in bones, promotes lipolysis (breakdown of fat tissue), and increases protein synthesis and muscle mass. Each of these effects is a powerful performance enhancer, and optimizing HGH levels is important for both athletes and anyone interested in exercise and high performance. Since the physiology of HGH is not well understood, however, it is important to optimize levels through natural methods.

Because HGH speeds recovery and regeneration, its use is banned by most sports organizations, including the International Olympic Committee. However, optimizing endogenous production of HGH (helping the body produce its own HGH) is not banned. Sleep stages 3 and 4 predominate in the first four or five hours of sleep. Optimizing sleep quality during this time can therefore maximize the amount of time spent in stages 3 and 4, and may help to provide the right conditions for natural growth-hormone release. Statistical data reveal that almost 40 million people in United States and Canada suffer from sleep disorders. Sleep should be a high priority, and we can take some immediate steps to improve it.

IMPROVING YOUR SLEEP

These tips should help you get a better night's sleep:

- ► Avoid caffeine 6 hours before you plan on sleeping.
- ► Finish your dinner 2 hours before sleeping.
- ► Avoid working or playing games on your computer just before dozing off.
- ► Create a stress-free environment by reading a book or listening to the radio. No screens.
- ► Exercising daily promotes sound sleep, but plan to stop exercise a couple of hours before bedtime.
- ► Keep the room temperature at 21°C. A cool bedroom gives a relaxed sleep.
- ► Go to bed before midnight. It promotes deeper sleep and better recovery.
- ► Avoid late-night snacks.
- ► Take a hot shower to relax. Research has shown that a rapid change in body temperature can help trigger drowsiness, so finish off your shower or bath with colder water.
- ► Develop your own sleep routine and then stay consistent.
- ► Sleep in as dark a room as possible.

If you have tried these tips and still have trouble sleeping (or your significant other thinks you're having trouble sleeping), consult your doctor. Additional medical tests and interventions can help.

Helpful links:

Centre for Sleep and Human Performance: www.centreforsleep.com

National Sleep Foundation: www.sleepfoundation.org

Human growth hormone affects many organs in ways that are not fully understood. Although doctors may prescribe this hormone (it has demonstrated benefits for patients with dwarfism, cardiac disease and growth disorders, and possibly in older people who are GH deficient), use by the general population is risky and should be avoided. For example, there is some research evidence that elevated levels of GH are associated with increased risks of some types of cancer.[60] It is thought that GH may hinder the processes in the body that kill off genetically damaged cells, and over the years this lack of action may accelerate cancer cell development and growth. It is important to note that research in this area is limited. I mention it to caution against using synthetic or supplemental growth hormone unless your doctor specifically recommends it.

MENSTRUAL CYCLE HORMONES AND EXERCISE PERFORMANCE

During adolescence, hormones are responsible for most of the profound physical changes that happen to all of us. Increased testosterone causes muscle tissue in boys to grow—hence, the physical change from boy to man. Estrogen and progesterone, secreted by the ovaries, are the hormones responsible for many of the changes in female physiology during adolescence, including the menstrual cycle.[61, 62]

Elite female athletes can take advantage of these hormones by aligning their training to their menstrual cycle. At different times of the cycle, endurance or strength capabilities may be increased or decreased, depending on estrogen or progesterone levels. For example, when these levels are both elevated, as in the mid-luteal phase (the part of the cycle that starts at ovulation and ends the day before the next period, usually 12–14 days), endurance performance may be improved. The increased amount of circulating estrogen acts on an enzyme called AMP kinase. This enzyme regulates metabolism in cells and affects mitochondrial function to improve energy production during exercise. But the improved endurance performance depends on there being more estrogen than progesterone, which is measured as the estrogen to progesterone ratio (E:P ratio). Progesterone is also a respiratory-system stimulant that acts on the peripheral chemoreceptors to increase sensitivity to oxygen and carbon dioxide levels. As I discussed in Chapter 1, breathing is a critical factor for exercise performance, so the respiratory effects of cycle hormones could explain some of the variations in performance that female athletes may experience over the course of a menstrual cycle.

Several groups of researchers have found that performance in all-out sprints and strength tests is best during menstruation. Carbohydrate metabolism is improved in the mid-follicular phase (the 10–16 days after menstruation). Since carbohydrates are the primary source of energy for the anaerobic system in the muscle, these results indicate that short-duration, high-intensity exercise performance may be increased in the mid-follicular phase.

The implications of these findings for athletes are that there may be benefits to controlling the menstrual cycle phase; for example, by using oral contraceptives to match the most beneficial phase to the time of the performance. Given that athletes must perform at a specific time and on a specific day, and this information is generally known months if not years in advance, adjusting the menstrual cycle is not difficult.

Another implication of these findings is that training or exercise plans can be aligned to match the menstrual cycle. This alignment allows for improved performance on a cyclic basis; the person undergoing exercise training would have an increased capacity for, and possibly responsiveness to, certain types of training at certain phases of the cycle. So, women reading this book could develop a plan that focuses on building strength and speed during menstruation by going to the gym and performing some strength and power workouts (see Chapter 2). Following menstruation, for about 10–14 days, there should be an increased focus on interval training and high-intensity, short-duration exercise. And then, in the last 10–16 days of the cycle, endurance exercise training should be emphasized. These examples show the importance of understanding how our bodies create and respond to hormone levels, because such awareness can help us to control our health and performance.

According to Dr. Jason Vescovi, research associate at Toronto's York University and sport scientist at the Canadian Sport Centre Ontario, the "female athlete triad" is a health condition with three interrelated components: energy balance, menstrual status and bone-mineral density. The consensus of the American College of Sports Medicine and the International Olympic Committee on what underlies the triad is something termed an energy deficit, or negative energy balance. An energy deficit occurs when physically active women do not consume enough calories to match their caloric expenditure, resulting in alterations to normal physiological functions.

We consume food that supplies the energy necessary to perform a wide range of physiological processes classified as essential (e.g., cellular maintenance), reducible (e.g., thermoregulation) or expendable (e.g., reproduction). The energy demands for a woman to ovulate every month are high and increase exponentially during pregnancy. Therefore, when the brain detects an energy deficit, a logical way to conserve energy is by shutting down the reproductive system, typically leading to overt signs of menstrual dysfunction such as irregular menses (oligomenorrhea) or absent menses (amenorrhea). In other words, this prevention of ovulation and, subsequently, of the chance of pregnancy, can be viewed as a protective mechanism against an even greater energy deficit and, in extreme cases, individual survival.

Menstrual dysfunction observed in association with an energy deficit has physiological implications. First, bone health in women is highly dependent on estrogen levels, and when the reproductive system shuts down, as in the case of the triad, these levels are suppressed, resulting in bone loss at a young age. A landmark study published in the *Journal of the American Medical Association* in 1990 by Dr. Barbara Drinkwater highlighted the strong relationship between menstrual history and bone health in young women.[63] Dr. Drinkwater's findings clearly demonstrate that women with a history of regular menstrual cycles also had the highest bone mineral density. Women with a history of absent or irregular menstrual cycles were found to have lower bone mineral density. Bone loss as a result of low estrogen levels is also commonly observed in post-menopausal women, but the subjects in this study were young, pre-menopausal women who exercised three or four days a week. Reductions in bone mineral density at a young age can result in greater fracture risk later in life.

Another implication of menstrual dysfunction observed with the triad is an increase in the potential for cardiovascular disease. Estrogen is believed to be cardio-protective—typically, an increased risk for cardio-vascular disease is observed in post-menopausal women. Recent evidence, however, indicates there are alterations in the vascular system, and markers of cardiovascular stress suggest that risks may also be greater in premenopausal women with suppressed levels of estrogen. Finally, there is also evidence that adaptations to training are attenuated in female athletes with menstrual dysfunction compared to those with normal menstruation, indicating that competitive athletes concerned with performance should at least be knowledgeable about the triad.

Treatment of women exhibiting the triad is a complex issue. Improving energy balance can help restore menstrual function, but the effects on bone health may not be completely reversible. Therefore, the education of coaches, parents and athletes is an important part of preventing the triad in young, physically active women.

WHAT HAPPENS WHEN THE ENDOCRINE SYSTEM BREAKS DOWN?

During my cycling trip through Africa, I learned a lot about what happens to the human body when it is pushed too far and when it does not work very well. About two-thirds of the way through the adventure, we were passing through southern Tanzania. It's a beautiful part of Africa, far from the tourist crowds around Mount Kilimanjaro and the Serengeti.

Unfortunately, I was still feeling the effects of drinking local water six weeks earlier in Ethiopia. I simply could not keep food in my digestive system for longer than 10 or 15 minutes. But I was also cycling 5 to 7 hours a day, burning energy from the limited amount of food I was able to eat. This situation produced a very interesting sensation (that's the scientist speaking, not the cyclist). As the foods or liquids I consumed entered my stomach, I could feel the sugars and fats enter my bloodstream and provide me with a surge of energy. This sensation usually lasted for about 30 to 45 minutes, and then I'd feel the opposite way—lethargic, heavy and drained. One day in Tanzania, my friend Steve Topham and I spent many hours riding together. Steve knew I was seriously fatigued and drained, and he was kind enough to let me ride my bike behind his so I could draft and have less air resistance to deal with. I was quite ill that day and had absolutely no energy. It was all I could do to keep pedalling the bike.

At about 2 p.m., after 6 hours of riding, we came across a little town and stopped for a break. A small store sold bottles of Coca-Cola. I drank one while a local boy in a Toronto Maple Leafs jersey stared at me. (I didn't have the energy to let him know that the Leafs had missed the playoffs again that year.) I felt this wonderful rush as the caffeine and sugar hit my bloodstream, setting in motion a cascade of events. First, as my blood sugar increased, β-cells of the islets of Langerhans in the pancreas (an organ that sits right below the stomach in the abdomen) released a hormone called insulin into my blood. Insulin acts on most tissues (the brain is the exception) to increase their absorption of glucose from the blood. Insulin attaches to a special receptor on the surface of the muscle cell or other target organ. The receptor communicates with a protein complex called GLUT-4. Insulin activates a signalling pathway that brings GLUT-4 transporters to the surface of the muscle. Once there, GLUT-4 pulls glucose from the blood into the muscle, where it is used to fuel metabolism. Because I was so energy-depleted on that ride, I could feel the sugars hit my bloodstream and then be absorbed into my muscles, where they supplied me with a surge of energy for about 30 minutes of cycling. Unfortunately, the energy quickly ran out, and I was soon hoping that Steve would continue to pull me along through the rest of the ride.

That day on the bike, I could feel the effects of insulin on my metabolism. But this insulin function sometimes fails, as it does in people with diabetes. There are two types of diabetes. In type 1 diabetes, also known as

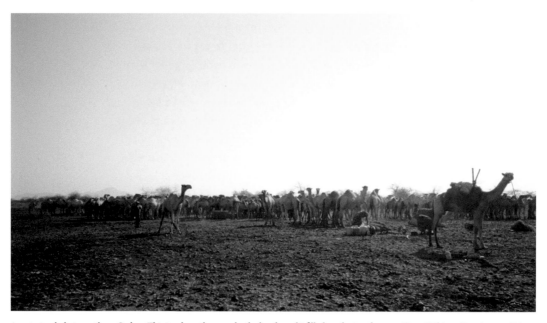

A watering hole in southern Sudan. This is where the camels, the locals and I filled up during the 2003 Tour d'Afrique bicycle expedition.

juvenile-onset diabetes, there is a deficiency of insulin and other hormones released from the pancreas. Metabolism then becomes fuelled by fats and proteins, a process that causes problems such as decreased circulation, nerve damage, susceptibility to infection, coma and, finally, death. This type of diabetes is difficult to treat and there is no absolute cure, only insulin injections. In type 2 diabetes, insulin production is relatively normal, but the receptor cells become desensitized to insulin. As a result, the target cells, such as the muscles or the liver, do not absorb glucose from the blood. This type of diabetes is associated with obesity and is closely related to lifestyle factors such as poor nutrition and lack of exercise. It can be managed through exercise and nutrition, which should be done under the supervision of a physician.

As for so many other chronic diseases, exercise can be used as therapy for both types of diabetes. Because exercise mimics the effects of insulin on blood-glucose levels and facilitates glucose uptake into the cells, it can help reduce the amount of insulin needed by type 1 diabetics. For type 2 diabetics, exercise can increase insulin sensitivity of the muscle tissue, thereby to some extent reversing the effects of the disease. According to the American Council on Exercise, individuals with diabetes should exercise at low-to-moderate intensity a minimum of 3 times per week, for about 20 to 60 minutes (under a doctor's care). Most aerobic activities are recommended for people with diabetes unless restricted because of medical complications. In addition to aerobic exercise, individuals with type 1 diabetes should engage in flexibility and strength-training exercises. Resistance training should also be performed at least 2 days per week, with a minimum of 1 set of 10 to 15 repetitions of each exercise at a low-to-moderate intensity. Safety precautions are necessary for people with diabetes, who should always consult a doctor before starting an exercise program.

There are some pretty inspirational stories of people performing at the elite world-class level despite having endocrine system problems such as diabetes. Gary Hall, Jr., is a U.S. swimmer who won eight Olympic medals in 1996 and 2000—four of them after having been diagnosed with type 2 diabetes in 1999. This achievement is even more incredible when you consider that Gary raced the 50- and 100-metre freestyle events. These last only 22 and 48 seconds, respectively, so energy production during these events relies mostly on anaerobic metabolism using glucose as fuel. Training for sprint events is extremely demanding, even for people with a healthy metabolism, and must have been incredibly challenging for Gary. In an interview with *Diabetes Health* in 2004, he described the effects of racing on his blood-glucose levels: "At the 2000 Olympics, I tested my blood glucose 10 minutes before my race, and it was 140 mg/dl. It was a 21-second race. Five minutes after the race, I tested again and it was 388 mg/dl. Then in 2004, before the Olympic trials in Long Beach, California, I tested 10 minutes before and it was 150 mg/dl. It was another 21-second race, and I qualified for the Olympics. Five minutes after the race, I tested, and it was 36 mg/dl. You never know what's going to happen. The only way to know is by testing." His story is inspirational because it shows that with great medical care, ongoing physiological testing and a commitment to health and training, anything is possible for people with diabetes.

The human endocrine system has a powerful impact on our health and performance. I believe that, by understanding how hormones affect our feelings, we can use our endocrine systems to live healthy, happy, product-ive lives. Research in this area is ongoing, and I am always excited to learn about new and interesting discoveries.

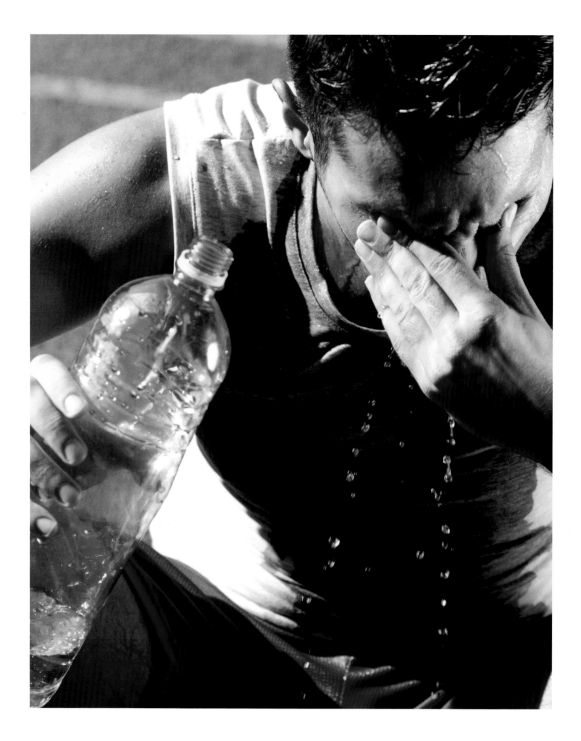

PERFORMANCE CYCLING
RECOVERY AND REGENERATION

6

Leading up to the 2000 Olympics in Sydney, Australia, I had the opportunity to work as a physiologist with the Canadian synchronized swimming team. "Synchro" is a sport that makes tremendous demands on an athlete. The swimmers have to be incredibly fit to perform a high-intensity routine that's four minutes long and requires near maximal oxygen uptake (VO_{2max}) cardiovascular system intensity, alternated with periods of extended breath-holding and explosive elements like jumps. Furthermore, the athletes need extraordinary flexibility, strength, balance, precision and timing, plus a myriad of other physical and mental skills to be able to compete effectively. I was amazed at the complexity of training—how these athletes got through eight-hour days of intense physical work. Typical days for these women consisted of water-based physical training, routine practice, ballet, stretching and weights, and land-based cardio. And this was done six days a week for the four years leading up to the Olympics, with only a couple of weeks a year for the athletes to take a break. The ability to recover within the day and between workouts defined the difference between those who could manage the training load and keep improving and those who couldn't and, ultimately, failed to qualify for the Olympics.

But hard training, work and practice cause mental and physical fatigue and distress—and stressors stimulate the body to adapt. The inductors that cause fatigue—for example, lactic acid, muscle-breakdown products such as creatine kinase, and neurotransmitters in the nerves—all stimulate the body to rebuild itself stronger. This adaptation also occurs in the brain, where new neural connections are made and neurotransmitter levels increase or decrease in response to the mental or physical training stimulus. But the real key to adaptation is the recovery period after the exercise is completed. This is when the refuelling, repair and growth of the body's systems take place. Train too hard, too often, and there won't be enough time for recovery. Instead of improving, the athlete deteriorates and gets sick.

Interestingly, the principles of recovery and regeneration apply to many disciplines beyond sport. Musicians need time to integrate the learning and practice periods before growth in their skills can take place. Similarly, businesspeople need time to recover after intense days in the boardroom, or following trips around the world to meet with colleagues. If physical or mental stress are maintained at too high a level for too long, deterioration in the musical or business performance will occur, just as it does in sports. Expose anyone to high levels of stress repeatedly without sufficient time to recover, and you'll have one exhausted and burned out executive, musician or athlete.

Constant fatigue or stress over time leads to a condition called over-reaching. Overreaching is a state where an individual's mental or physical performance is compromised. Simply put, they are too tired to perform well. But if adequate rest is provided for someone in the overreaching state, then the condition is easily reversed. If, for example, you work really hard all week so that by Friday afternoon you're exhausted and mentally fatigued, a great weekend of rest and relaxation can bring you back to 100% by Monday morning.

Overtraining is more serious. According to the *Oxford Dictionary of Sports Science and Medicine*, overtraining is a complex syndrome, described as "a combination of signs and symptoms, which cause the sufferer to feel mentally fatigued in absence of physical fatigue with a deterioration of performance." [64]

Overtraining occurs when athletes perform high-volume or high-intensity training consistently over time without allowing for adequate recovery. Performance becomes compromised, and unlike the overreaching state, it is not easily reversible by rest. In fact, it may take many months of complete rest to bring the athlete back to a point where the body can begin to adapt positively to a physical training challenge. Although overtraining is a term used mostly in the context of athletics, I think that the same problem exists in the working world. One has only to look at the rates of chronic

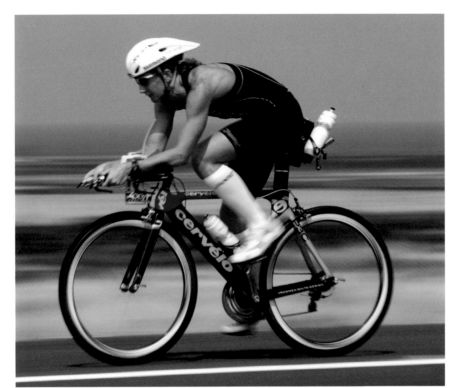

Ironman triathlete Tara Norton wearing compression gear on her lower legs during the Hawaii Ironman World Championships.

fatigue, cardiovascular disease, depression and long-term disability in our society to realize that overtraining is happening all around us. This concept may be the most important area of overlap of sports and business, where sports can have a powerful impact on our world by helping all of us to understand how to recover and regenerate so that our health and performance improve over time.

I don't think that high-performance requirements or time pressures are going to disappear in either sports or business. So the challenge is to determine how to maximize our adaptation and improvement so we remain healthy, both mentally and physically. That can be done by (1) ensuring there is enough low-stress rest time between work or training sessions to allow for recovery to occur, or (2) speeding recovery and regeneration so that the individual has adapted optimally before the beginning of the next training session. The first option is acceptable if there are no time constraints on the learning curve or the expected improvement. For example, if someone is trying to improve their health by running, then providing

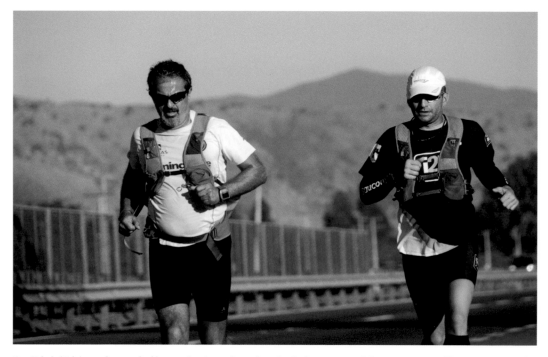

Ray Zahab (right) ran almost a double marathon in 40-degree heat, but he has a unique ability to recover quickly. A common mistake athletes make is to put too much emphasis on training and not enough on recovery.

adequate time for recovery between sessions is excellent. This recovery time will allow the individual to improve and the body to adapt. This option would also apply to anyone who is learning a new instrument as a hobby. But it is not an adequate method if there are time pressures for improvement. In most cases, athletes are interested in improving as quickly as possible—in which case we have to try speeding recovery and regeneration.

If we can maximize the rate of recovery after a workout or stressor, then the body and brain will continue to improve over many years. Ultimately, this process is the key to performance excellence in any discipline. And the great thing is that the techniques used by world-class athletes to optimize recovery are available to anyone.

I'll show you these techniques as a timeline: from what to do immediately after a stressor, up to what can be done hours after the workout. Although I'll talk about athletes and workouts and training, the techniques can be applied to nearly any situation. I'll also distinguish between physical and mental recovery and regeneration where necessary, although in many cases they're linked. Let's start with what can be done to improve performance immediately.

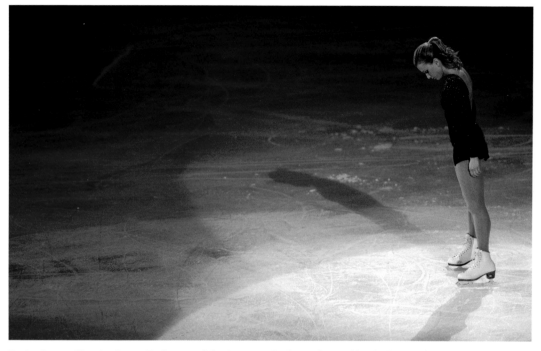

During the 2010 Olympics, Joannie Rochette nearly lost her nerve after her mother's sudden death. But before her performance, under incredible pressure, she applied breathing techniques and went on to win a bronze medal.

STEP 1: INSTANT RESPONSE

Breathe!

A moment that caught the world's imagination during the 2010 Winter Olympics in Vancouver was the performance of Joannie Rochette during her short skate program after her mother died suddenly only days before. People were amazed by Joannie's nearly flawless performance on the ice. However, I think the critical performance-enhancing moment occurred before the music even started. As Joannie skated onto the ice to assume her start position, the crowd began cheering loudly. At that moment, she began to become emotional and lose focus and control. She had the composure to turn around, return to the side of the ice, take a drink of water and then take three deep, slow breaths before returning to the ice to begin her performance. This was a brilliant move that allowed her to release some physical tension through a breathing technique, and also to recover her mental focus to stay concentrated on skating and skating only.

I used exactly the same breathing technique in my first on-camera interview of the Olympic coverage when I spoke about the tragic events

RELAXATION BREATHING TECHNIQUE

You can perform relaxation breathing by expanding your abdomen so that your stomach rises with every inhalation and lowers when you exhale. Try to slow the breathing down to six seconds in and six seconds out. This exercise, which can be performed at any time, has immediate benefits.

This technique is a key skill for athletes, professional musicians, business professionals and anyone else who has to perform under pressure. Imagine taking just seconds to compose yourself before starting a key presentation or stepping onto the stage to perform a recital. Imagine if we did this right before walking into our homes at the end of a brutally stressful day. Take just a moment to relax, let go and focus on the important task at hand rather than on the past or future. It's a very powerful technique. The applications for this are endless. Deep breathing is a great tool for relaxing the body and letting the stressful moment go so you can focus and concentrate on your next performance. Try it out the next time you are feeling anxious, nervous or stressed.

at the sliding track on Day 1, when Nodar Kumaritashvili, the Lithuanian luger, was killed during a training run. As the lights came on and we sat in the studio waiting for the broadcast to start, the accident was replayed for us. Watching the horrific crash was brutally emotional. Added to this was the nervousness I felt, given that I had done live TV on only a few occasions before the Olympics and never for an audience like the one I was about to address. I was nervous. And as physiologist, I was able to recognize the effect my mental stress was having on my body. (This ability is a possible downside of knowing a lot about the human body. You are fully aware of what is happening to you in crisis moments: the shaking hands, the dry mouth and, basically, the full sympathetic nervous system response and all the feelings you don't want to have when you're about to do a live interview in front of millions of people.) Fortunately, when a colleague spoke for the first minute of the live interview, I took three deep, slow breaths. The effects on me physically and mentally were powerful. My body relaxed, I stopped shaking, saliva returned to my mouth and throat so I could speak, and most importantly, I was able to think clearly to answer the questions related to the accident.

An inspirational performance like Joannie Rochette's provides a powerful lesson. But I think that our knowledge of human physiology can help us take it a step further. Understanding the physiological effects provides a rationale for actually implementing these techniques, because we know that they work for all of us—not just super humans like Olympians. Take deep breathing for example. When we get nervous or stressed out, we resort to short, fast, shallow breaths. This pattern ventilates the top part of our lungs—eliminating carbon dioxide and oxygenating our blood so that our muscles and brains get the fuel they need for moving and thinking.

Unfortunately, this shallow-breathing reaction does not work very well for us because it exchanges air only in the upper parts of the lungs. The problem is that the blood passing through our lungs is a liquid. And because all liquids are subject to gravity, the majority of the blood is pulled into the lower parts of the lungs, which are not as well ventilated as the upper portions. The deep-breathing technique exchanges oxygen and carbon dioxide throughout most of the lungs and therefore may increase the oxygenation of the blood. The fuels available at that moment for a mental and physical performance will, in turn, be increased as well.

In addition to improving gas exchange, deep breathing can also lower your body's overall tension, both physically and mentally. The actual physiological link here has not been proven because it is very hard to do brain studies in humans, but I have a hypothesis based on some interesting research that my PhD supervisor, Dr. James Duffin from the University of Toronto's Respiratory Research Group, performed. Dr. Duffin is interested in the control of breathing, and, as part of his research, he and his graduate students used rats to map neurones in the brain stem which control the diaphragm muscle (the big muscle that passes across the abdomen and is responsible for inhalation). Dr. Duffin and his colleagues studied an area of the brain stem containing many different groups of neurones involved in controlling breathing. These nerve centres are all interconnected to form a neural network. Similarly, there are clusters of neurones in the brain stem controlling the heart and the sympathetic nervous system. These controlling centres are interlinked and are affected by the signals that pass between the brain and the body. Most of us cannot control our heart and sympathetic nervous system directly, but we can control our breathing. I hypothesize that, by gaining control of the signals

GREG'S HIGH-PERFORMANCE TIPS

TENSION RELEASE

"Bracing" is a term that describes the tightening and tensing of muscles—you feel it when you lift your eyebrows or raise your shoulders. People can get tense when they are tired or nervous. Practising tension release can break the bracing habit and lead to muscle relaxation and faster swimming through improved circulation and improved energy levels. Tension release involves becoming aware of muscle tightness and body position. You can build such awareness by consistently asking yourself several questions:

- ► Can I drop my shoulders?
- ► Can I relax my hands? Stomach? Legs? Forehead?
- ► Can I sit in a more comfortable position?
- ► Can I relax and deepen my breathing?

Try to recognize when an area of your body is tense, and then release the tension from your muscles and let go of the tightness.

activating in the breathing neurones of the medulla, we can also calm the nerve centres for other autonomic functions controlling the heart and sympathetic nervous system, thereby affecting intensity of traffic from the body to the brain, and vice versa. This hypothesis may be the physiological explanation for why deep breathing can calm the body and the brain under the most challenging circumstances.

Rehydrate

A critical factor for recovery during or post-workout, and perhaps the most important one, is rehydrating. We all know that we sweat when we participate in sports or exercise. We sweat in order to remove heat from our bodies, but water is also consumed within the cell itself. When we break down fuels such as carbohydrates, proteins and fats for energy, the body uses water in the process, specifically in the mitochondria (the energy-producing structures inside your cells). Many of the vitamins the body employs are dissolved in water for transportation and other uses. In fact, water is used in most cellular processes. This may be why we can survive for only a few days without water, and why our bodies are 60% water. Decreases in hydration can cause decreases in plasma volume (the fluid part of your blood), making it harder for the heart to pump blood. A decrease of 1 to 2% hydration has been shown to lower muscle performance, and, disturbingly, this decrease in hydration is typical for a 90-minute to 2-hour workout, which most athletes complete daily. Decreasing hydration also has a negative impact on cognitive function. This makes hydration critical for sports where decision-making is important (or for people who want to be able to think clearly in the afternoon at work).

Finding the right amount of fluid to drink during and after exercise is highly individual and depends on the type and intensity of the workout. In general, we recommend drinking 1 litre of fluid for each kilogram of weight lost during exercise. We also recommend water for any training session lasting up to one hour, and then sports drinks for training or competition lasting longer than that. We also suggest monitoring hydration levels by paying attention to the colour of urine. A large amount of light-coloured, diluted urine probably means you are hydrated; dark-coloured, concentrated urine probably means you are dehydrated.

It's important to pay attention to the issue of hydration because even the most experienced international-level athletes can improve their

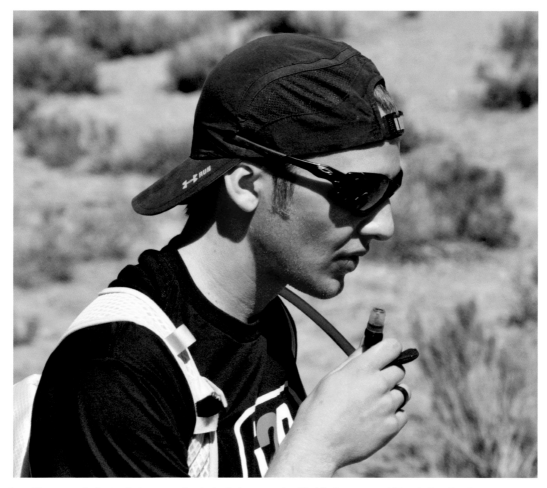
Ryan Montgomery hydrating during a marathon in the Andes mountains. We dehydrate more quickly at higher altitudes.

hydration practices. Adam McKillop, a graduate student who worked with me while completing his master's degree in exercise physiology, made a very interesting discovery by accident. As part of his research project, Adam was tracking the hydration levels of swimmers during training sessions at both sea level and altitude. (Altitude is a factor that increases the risk of dehydration.) He was also working on developing a sports drink mix to meet the exact fluid, sugar and electrolyte needs of the athletes we were working with. Adam measured the specific gravity and osmolality (the number of particles in a fluid) of urine samples from the athletes before and after practice to determine if the sports drink was helping to manage the dehydration that accumulated during practice. It turned out that the

GREG'S HIGH-PERFORMANCE TIPS

STAY HYDRATED DURING EXERCISE

During a workout, drink 250 to 500 millilitres of liquid per hour. Drink water during workouts of up to 90 minutes, and sports drinks if practice is longer. For after training, I recommend drinking 1 litre per 1 kilogram of body weight lost.

drink worked very well. In fact, it worked so well that hydration levels actually improved during workout, despite the fact that the athletes were exercising intensely for two hours. This observation led us to an interesting conclusion—the athletes were showing up to workout dehydrated. They would do a great job of drinking during practice from 6 a.m. to 8 a.m. and from 4 p.m. to 6 p.m., but neglected to stay hydrated in the intervening hours, when they were at school. Staying hydrated requires constant attention. Our discovery probably applies to most people, who don't drink enough water during the day to stay healthy and perform at their best.

STEP 2: IMMEDIATELY AFTER TRAINING

Cool-Down (Active Recovery)

Most people have heard that it is important to "cool down" after a workout. Well, for athletes it is critical. I've had the opportunity to work as an exercise physiologist at major international competitions, mostly in the sport of swimming. During competition, athletes produce tremendous amounts of lactic acid because of the high intensity of the exercise. In most sports, an event is rarely won in a single race. Many events require athletes to perform heats, semi-finals and finals on their way to a possible medal. Also, in many cases athletes perform in more than one event, or may have their individual events and then also team events such as relays. Of course, the ultimate example of recovery is Michael Phelps, who swam 17 times on his way to winning eight gold medals in a single Olympics. So, removing metabolic by-products as quickly as possible after racing is important; it ensures the athlete starts the next event in a rested state. The primary role of the physiologist during actual competition is helping the athletes recover as quickly as possible by optimizing the "cool-downs" or, as I prefer to call it, "active recovery."

Removing metabolic waste quickly has been shown to improve the speed of glycogen re-synthesis. Basically, if you leave lactate in the muscle, the mitochondria have to keep working to process the lactate. If you recover passively by resting, which feels really good, especially after a hard race, then the rate of lactate removal from muscle is extremely slow—in the order of hours. However, counter to what you may think, exercising at

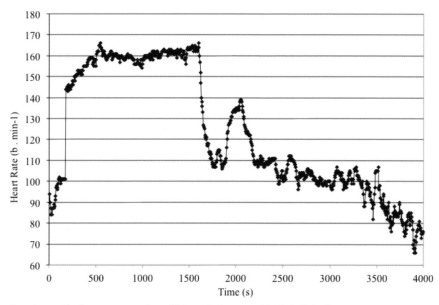

A good example of a proper warm-down. This graph shows an athlete's declining heart rate.

a low-to-moderate intensity actually speeds up the removal of metabolic waste products like lactic acid. And as soon as the muscle and blood lactic-acid levels are back to baseline, the muscle can start using glucose to restock its energy stores, ensuring that when the athletes start the next race they have a full tank of muscle fuel.

Dr. Argyris Toubekis, from the Democritus University of Thrace in Greece, conducted a study in which swimmers completed a 100-metre time trial. They then either rested for 15 minutes or performed 5 minutes of light exercise at 60% of their maximum heart rates and then rested for 10 minutes. Fifteen minutes after the initial time trial, the athletes completed a second time trial. The athletes who performed the 5 minutes of active recovery swam 1.4 seconds faster than when they simply rested. So for athletes who have to perform multiple events in a single day, or are involved in competitions where they are required to perform on several occasions over a tournament, I suggest active recovery after each performance.

The question then becomes how to optimize the removal of waste products. This is accomplished by having athletes exercise at the highest intensity, for which there is no lactate production by the muscles. This procedure ensures that the amount of blood flow circulating through the body is maximized, but with minimal anaerobic stress on the metabolism of the muscle. The body is then better able to circulate the lactic acid from the muscle fibres that produce it (our type IIs) to the muscle fibres that can use lactate as fuel (the type Is).

To exercise in this target zone, you can estimate your maximum heart rate by subtracting 0.85 times your age from 217:

$$\textit{Maximum heart rate} = 217 - \underline{\hspace{1cm}} (0.85 \times \textit{your age}) = \underline{\hspace{1cm}} \textit{beats/minute (b/m)}$$

Dr. W.C. McMaster, from the University of Virginia, has determined that active recovery at 55 to 65% of maximum intensity is the most effective way to enhance the clearance of blood lactate after exercise.[65] His study was conducted on university-level athletes; therefore, for the non-athlete (but still active individual), we recommend decreasing the active recovery intensity to between 50 and 55% of maximum. You can implement this intensity by taking your maximum heart rate and multiplying by 0.50 to 0.55.

Now you know the work-intensity heart rate you need to remove waste products after your workout. The next question that I'm always asked by athletes during active recovery is "How long to I have to do this for?" The answer depends on the intensity of the exercise you just finished. My research team analyzed the lactate clearance rates of 100 athletes after races to determine how much active recovery was needed following competition.[66] We found that, in general, it takes about 1 minute of active recovery to clear 1 mmol/L of blood lactate. So we now have the following recommendations for active recovery times after exercise:

EXERCISE TIME	ESTIMATED BLOOD-LACTATE LEVEL	RECOMMENDED RECOVERY TIME
30 seconds	6–8 mmol/L	6–8 minutes
1 minute	10–16 mmol/L	10–16 minutes
2 minutes	10–16 mmol/L	10–16 minutes
4 minutes	8–12 mmol/L	8–12 minutes
8–15 minutes	6–8 mmol/L	6–8 minutes
30–60 minutes	4–6 mmol/L	10 minutes*
Strength training	6–10 mmol/L	15 minutes**

* Longer aerobic sessions are physiologically stressful in ways that are not always related to blood-lactate concentration. To ensure adequate clearance of all waste products, recover for 10 minutes at light intensity following any interval of cardio workout.

** Similarly, during weights sessions, the stress on muscle fibres is significant. To ensure adequate clearance of waste products, we recommend active recovery at 50 to 55% of maximum heart rate for at least 10 minutes.

Refuel

Exercise training takes energy supplied through the breakdown of carbohydrates and fats. During most types of training, our muscles are placed under tremendous stress, which stimulates the body to rebuild itself. Most structures in the body are made of proteins. Research clearly shows that refuelling the body immediately after exercise with carbohydrates[67] and proteins speeds the replenishment of energy stores and protein synthesis and reduces muscle inflammation and soreness.[68] Carbohydrates are critical for replenishing muscle glycogen stores, and proteins are crucial for initiating muscle and other soft-tissues repair. The question is, how much of each should you consume? In part, the answer depends on the type of exercise you performed. Endurance athletes such as cyclists, triathletes, runners and swimmers exercise longer at sustained intensities. This type of work depletes muscle glycogen, so replenishing it is a priority. Without enough glycogen they can't work at high intensities, or they may run out of fuel in their next training session. Therefore, for endurance athletes we recommend consuming a light snack with a ratio of 4 carbohydrates to 1 protein. Check out the box for some post-workout snack ideas.

Strength training or sports that require greater demands on muscles produce micro-tears in the muscle and soft tissues such as tendons or capillary beds. For any exercise that makes your muscles sore, protein synthesis is therefore crucial to repair these tissues. In this case, the ratios change, and a higher protein content is warranted. We recommend about 2:1 carbohydrates to proteins after a strength-type workout. As little as 6 to 10 grams of protein accelerate protein synthesis in the muscles follow-ing exercise, but you can calculate your approximate protein requirement based on your body weight. In general, sedentary people need about 0.8 grams of protein per kilogram of body weight, and active people

WHAT'S THE BEST SNACK BAR FOR POST-WORKOUT RECOVERY?

What's the best choice for a cardio workout or a weight-training session? The key to picking the right post-workout snack is to check the carbohydrate-to-protein ratio. Here are a few examples:

▸ *Power Bar Protein Plus.* 300 calories, 37 g carb, 24 g protein. 1.5 carbs to protein. Good for post-strength training workout.

▸ *Power Bar Recovery.* 260 calories, 30 g carb, 12 g protein. 3:1 carbs to protein. Good for interval workout or circuits in the gym.

▸ *Lara Bar.* 240 calories, 23 g carb, 6 g protein. 4:1 carbs to protein. Good for after cardio workout.

▸ *Clif Bar.* 250 calories, 46 g carb, 11 g protein. 4+:1 carbs to protein. Good for during cardio exercise.

▸ *Life Sport Zone.* 300 calories, 39 g carb, 24g protein. 2:1 carbs to protein. Good for after strength-training session.

▸ *Almonds* (50 grams, 1/3 cup). 320 calories, 10 g carb, 10 g protein. 1:1 carbs to protein + lots of fat. Excellent snack for midday between meals. Provides long-term energy that prevents crashes.

need much more—about 1.6 to 1.8 grams per kilogram. Regular foods (e.g., chicken, beef, fish, beans and legumes, and eggs) can provide the necessary amino acids, and some protein powders are acceptable and convenient options.

Carbohydrates are the fuels our muscles need to perform at a high level. In the body, the carbohydrate foods we eat are broken down into smaller components like glucose, or are stored as more complex molecules like glycogen. Research indicates that athletes should consume carbohydrates within the first 30 minutes following exercise to optimize replacement of muscle glycogen stores.[69] When we eat carbohydrates, the body responds by releasing insulin, which helps the muscles, the liver and the brain to absorb glucose from the blood. Simple carbohydrates that break down quickly (like white bread or raw sugar), causing a rapid increase in blood-sugar levels and correspondingly producing a surge in insulin levels, are called high–glycemic index foods. (For more information, check out the brilliant book *The GI Diet* at www.gidiet.com.) Complex carbohydrates (e.g., whole-wheat bread or wild or brown rice) break down slowly and produce smaller changes in blood-glucose levels, and therefore are called low–glycemic index foods.

It is hard to know what kind of carbohydrate to eat right after a workout to speed fuel replenishment.[70] I've developed some simple rules for my athletes that help determine what type of carbohydrate to use, and when. Basically, the closer the next exercise bout, the more you can rely on simple carbohydrates. For example, during a basketball game simple carbohydrates are the best option because you are trying to keep blood-glucose levels high. In this case, a sports drink would be a good option. If you have to perform another exercise within a couple of hours, such as during a tennis tournament, then carbohydrates that are easy to digest are your best bet. In this case, a whole-wheat bagel would be a good option. But if the next training or competition session is more than a few hours away, then you should rely on complex carbohydrates, proteins and even some fats to supply a sustained level of consistent energy, and nutrients to help rebuild body tissues.

There is an optimal time window for refuelling, and again research suggests that eating within 30 minutes of finishing exercise is critical. After this 30-minute window, the muscles shut down and won't absorb any new nutrients for as long as a few hours; the muscles become insensitive to insulin, the hormone that signals cells to absorb glucose from the bloodstream. In other words, eating an hour after you finish practice will not help speed recovery. For athletes, this timing is critical because they are often trying to perform at a very high level every 12 hours—basically morning and evening workouts. Preparing for the next session depends on getting refuelled and repaired as quickly as possible. I believe that this refuelling applies to people who like to exercise in the morning before going to work. If you exercise in the morning and don't replenish your muscle energy early on, then throughout the morning your muscles and brain will compete for precious energy resources in the form of blood glucose. Your muscles use glucose to replenish their glycogen stores, and your brain uses glycogen to fuel the neural activity that's required for thinking, memory processing and other functions. So the post-workout meal is important not only for athletes who have to worry about training at a high level consistently, but also for people with multiple high-performance demands.

STEP 3: REDUCE INFLAMMATION OR STIMULATE ADAPTATION

Athletes push themselves to the limit as often as possible. They do long endurance-training sessions, where the aerobic system is maxed out for hours; anaerobic interval training, where high intensity is mixed with lower-intensity recovery; and strength-training sessions, where

<aside>

⚜ GREG'S HIGH-PERFORMANCE TIPS

CARBOHYDRATES ARE THE PRIMARY FUELS FOR MUSCLES AND THE BRAIN

Carbohydrates supply the body's immediate energy needs as well as fuels for replenishment of muscle glycogen. Carbohydrate recommendations for athletes range from 5 to 12 g/kg per day. Athletes engaged in low-intensity training can consume lower amounts of carbohydrates (5 to 7 g/kg/d). During moderate-to-heavy training, higher carbohydrate intake is acceptable (7 to 10 g/kg/d). Anyone doing extreme aerobic exercise (four to six hours a day) can consume 10 to 12 g/kg/d.

Source: Burke, 2006.

</aside>

the muscles are put under so much pressure they literally tear at the microscopic level. So far in this chapter, I've talked about recovery techniques that deal mostly with removing waste products formed during the training session, and with refuelling the body with sugars for energy and proteins for rebuilding and adaptation. But the rebuilding and adaptation process takes more work and time than simply removing lactic acid from the muscle and blood (minutes) and replenishing muscle glucose and glycogen (minutes to hours). Until very recently, we thought that the faster you could return the body to its baseline homeostasis point, the better—because this condition was most conducive to the next training session. This process involved applying techniques to minimize inflammation in the body as quickly as possible. But recent research has highlighted how helpful tissue inflammation is in stimulating the body to rebuild itself to be stronger.

When muscle fibres are damaged—for example, after a hard weights session when your muscles are sore—inflammatory cells rush to the area to clean up the damaged tissue and stimulate new fibres to regenerate. These inflammatory cells are called macrophages. They are present in the blood, and when a tissue is injured these cells are often first on the scene. The macrophages literally eat up the damaged tissues. Gaps in the damaged cell walls open, allowing fluids to rush in and causing inflammation and swelling. Meanwhile, the inflammatory process stimulates production of a substance called insulin-like growth factor-1 (IGF-1). This powerful hormone circulates through the body and works on areas such as damaged muscle fibres that have been cleaned up by macrophages. The IGF-1 signals growth cells in the muscle tissue (called satellite cells) to build new muscle fibres and repair damaged ones. The end result is newer, stronger and more numerous muscle fibres. A similar process occurs when tendons are damaged. The benefit of this process is that it stimulates new and stronger tissues. The drawback is that it is very painful, and it takes some time for this process to run its natural course.

In fact, the healing process I've just described can take as much as 72 hours for muscles or even longer for tendons and other soft tissues. Most of the time, athletes don't have this long—they usually have at least two practice sessions a day. So we are currently attempting a balanced approach. We allow healing to occur on its own as often as possible, but if the athlete is in competition, or absolutely has to have another quality practice session within 12 to 24 hours, then we use techniques like cold therapy or compression clothing to reduce inflammation as quickly as possible.

If an athlete has to perform again in a short time—within 24 hours—then the objective of the recovery process will be to speed healing so that the body is ready to go as soon as it can. If this is the case, then reducing inflammation is the key. And the best way to do this is ... an ice bath. Yes, that's correct: not a nice warm relaxing soak in the tub, but a short dip in water that has been cooled to between 12 and 15°C. (Warning: if the water is too cold, it can cause tissue damage. American sprinter Justin Gatlin gave himself frostbite three weeks before world championships in the summer of

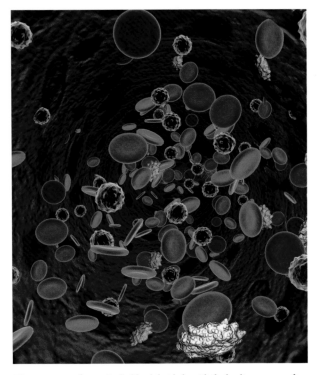

There are many factors in the blood that help with the healing process after exercise.

2011. If you want to try this technique, keep the water temperature above 12°c.) Ice baths cause blood vessels to constrict,[71] forcing waste products out of the affected area. It's almost like wringing out a sponge. When the area warms up again, new blood rushes in to help the healing process. Or at least that's the theory.

Although many athletes swear by this technique, research is less conclusive. Recently a team in the United Kingdom tested whether 10 minutes of immersion in cold water would improve recovery from exercise-induced muscle damage.[72] Volunteers performed 10 sets of 10 plyometric vertical jumps to cause muscle damage. The scientists assessed the enzyme creatine kinase (a marker of muscle breakdown), muscle soreness and muscle strength at several intervals after the jumps and found no differences between athletes who received the ice bath and those who did not. This research suggests that total body immersion in cold water may not help muscles recover from severe exercise. But a different study, from the Université de Picardie Jules Verne in France, conducted similar research measuring the effect of cold-water immersion on the nervous system.[73] The French researchers examined measures of heart-rate variability, which tests the regularity of the heartbeat and is thought to reflect the activation of the parasympathetic nervous system. The more regular and even the heartbeat, the more relaxed the nervous system is. The researchers determined that water immersion increased parasympathetic (the "rest and recovery") nervous system activity, and that colder water enhanced this response. Another group of French researchers found that cold-water immersion after exhaustive anaerobic sprint exercise kept levels of inflammatory markers like leukocytes (blood cells that are produced to help clean up tissue damage in the body) lower than immersion in temperate water. The reduced levels of inflammation led to a more rapid recovery in terms of anaerobic exercise performance.[74]

Research indicates that cold-water immersion may not help muscles recover from plyometric exercise. However, it does seem to reduce inflammation and improve nervous-system function to facilitate the processes in the body that are governed by the parasympathetic nervous system (e.g., digestion and circulation). The best support for the effectiveness of this technique comes from the large numbers of athletes who continue to use cold-water immersion—athletes and their coaches are often years ahead of researchers in figuring out what works best for improving human performance and health. For example, Peter Brukner of the University of Melbourne, one of the researchers who published results that show no benefits for recovery of muscle strength after cold therapy, said in an interview with *The Globe and Mail* that "Even though our research [on ice baths] was unconvincing, I still encourage their use." Most readers of this book won't have access to an ice bath but can still take advantage of this technique. The simplest thing to do is to have a very cold shower or bath after exercising. Make sure that you keep the water flowing on an area of your skin until it is cold to the touch, and that you cover as much of your body as possible. Try to keep this up for about 5 minutes—this should activate your parasympathetic nervous system and speed your recovery from your workout.

COMPRESSION GARMENTS

A tool in the athlete's arsenal for speeding recovery has recently gained popularity: wearing very tight compression garments. The current generation of such compression gear has its roots in the treatment of medical conditions such as blood clots or peripheral circulatory disease. Doctors found that wearing compression socks improved blood flow from the periphery back to the heart. Compression socks or arm garments are designed to become tighter the farther away from the heart; for example, they're tighter around the ankle than the knee. Athletes often wear compression garments or sports tights after training sessions. A group of scientists had volunteers perform 10 sets of 10 plyometric jumps to induce muscle damage and soreness.[75] Half the volunteers wore compression garments on their legs for 12 hours. All the participants returned to the lab the next day for retesting. Interestingly, those who wore the compression pants had less of a decrement in their ability to jump—the non-compression group could jump only 85% of their height from the previous day, while the compression group was able to reach 95% of their initial test results. The compression group also reported less muscle soreness, but there were no differences in the levels of creatine kinase (an enzyme that's associated with of muscle damage) between the two groups.

Imagine the impact such a tool could have on a sport like volleyball, which demands explosive jumps repeatedly during a game and over the several days that make up a tournament. Furthermore, the more successful teams are, the more they have to play—and the more explosive jumping they do. The same can be said for other court-based sports like basketball. But again, the recently discovered advantage is that using this gear reduces inflammation and swelling. This is great if you have to compete again in a matter of hours, but highly problematic if you want to stimulate the body to adapt positively over the long term. So, while the gear can be helpful in competition, or during a critical high-intensity training block, it should not be used regularly.

However, it appears that compression gear does not improve endurance performance. Some experts have suggested that compression gear could act like an extra pump, improving blood flow through the veins and back to the heart. Three research studies tested the effects of compression gear on cycling[76] and running,[77, 78] and none showed that performance was improved. So for now it looks like using compression gear for recovery after

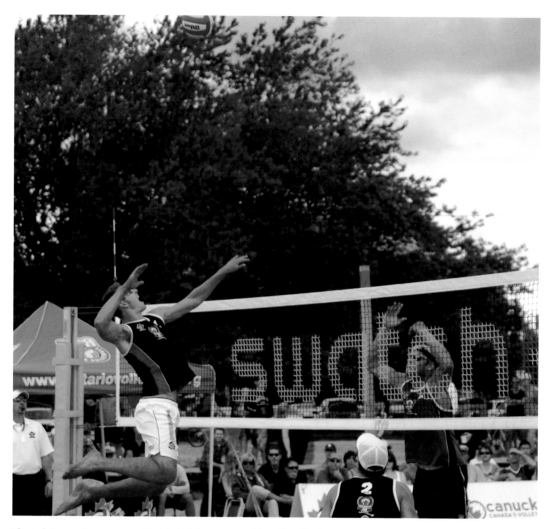

Physical stress makes recovery critical for high-impact sports like volleyball, where repeated explosive jumping can damage muscles, joints and nerves.

muscle-damaging exercise is the way to go, but only if you have to perform at a high level again within a relatively short time frame.

MASSAGE

Everyone I know loves a good massage. Athletes are heavy users of massage therapy, especially at major games. I think that, if given the choice, most would prefer to have their massage therapist with them at the Olympics over every other type of sport science or sports medicine practitioner. The research supporting the use of massage therapy is less than conclusive, but if we apply our inflammation theory to this discipline, an understanding of how massage can help athletes, and the rest of us, emerges quite clearly.

In the past it was thought that massage helped speed recovery from exercise by "flushing out" our muscle tissue and thereby speeding the removal of lactic acid after exercise. Some recent work by Michael Tschakovsky, an associate professor in the School of Kinesiology and Health Studies at Queen's University in Kingston, Ontario, has shown this is probably not the case.[79] Dr. Tschakovsky asked his research volunteers to squeeze a handgrip for 2 minutes at 40% of their maximum. This action produces huge amounts of lactic acid in the forearm muscles and is quite painful. The researchers then collected blood samples from the vein that drains the forearm muscles, and tested whether passive rest, light muscle contractions at 10% of maximum, or massage of the forearm muscles was most effective at removing lactic acid and improving blood flow through the muscles. Surprisingly, massage decreased blood flow. Each stroke blocked blood flow to the tissues, and also decreased the rate of lactic-acid removal.

But there are aspects of massage therapy other than lactate removal. Further research has shown that massage therapy decreases levels of cortisol (the hormone associated with the stress response). And most people report feeling better and more recovered after a massage. Reduced muscle soreness and decreased inflammation may therefore be the biological mechanism that explains why people swear by massage therapy. Some new research on rabbits actually backs up this idea.[80] It showed that massaged muscle regained 59% of strength lost due to a severe exercise bout after four days, whereas rested muscles regained only 14%. The massaged muscles had few of the inflammatory markers associated with muscle damage, and also

> ### ✦ GREG'S HIGH-PERFORMANCE TIPS
>
> #### HOW ATHLETES USE MASSAGE THERAPY
> *Pre-event*
> Involves light, rapid strokes that work as part of a warm-up to increase blood flow, loosen muscles and activate the nervous system. Often done over clothing.
> *Post-event*
> Involves slower, more relaxing strokes, moving from distal toward the heart to encourage tissue drainage. May also help move fluid through the lymphatic system.
> *During training*
> Known more commonly as "sport massage," this is deep-tissue massage that's often quite uncomfortable. Helpful in the treatment of injuries and for decreasing muscle tension patterns.

weighed less. This finding suggests that there may have been less damage to the muscle fibre membranes, thereby reducing overall and intra-fibre swelling. The authors of the study could not discern whether the results were due to a decreased inflammatory response immediately after the exhaustive exercise bout or due to more rapid tissue healing.

Brand new studies by Dr. Mark Tarnopolsky's research group at McMaster University has confirmed these findings in humans. Graduate student Justin Crane found that, despite not having an effect on lactate or glycogen levels, massage decreased inflammatory markers and cellular stress[81]. It appears that massage therapy is not ideal for lactic acid removal, but is excellent for reducing tissue inflammation and physiological markers of stress.

THE RECOVERY FLOW CHART

The following steps may seem like a lot to apply, but by adhering to them you can radically improve your health and performance at any level—from someone just starting a running program right through to an Olympic champion. Try this system out the next time you finish a practice, and you'll be amazed at the difference it makes. If you can do these steps consistently, this program can revolutionize your health and recovery.

After a workout, race or high-stress event

1   Breathe: 60 seconds slow, deep breathing.
2   Rehydrate: 1 litre water/1 kilogram body-weight lost.
3   Recover: 1 minute/1 mmol of lactate, or 5 minutes after an easy workout; 10 minutes after a moderate session; 15 minutes after hard training.
4   Refuel: Eat a carbohydrate and protein snack within 30 minutes.
    If there is another performance event within 48 hours then complete steps 5 and 6, if not go to step 7.
5   Take a cold bath or shower: 5 minutes on, 5 minutes off (× 2).
6   Wear your compression gear for 2 or 3 hours.
    (Note: If you are getting tired or run down, you can do steps 5 and 6 any time.)
7   Get a weekly massage. Check out a local massage school—the prices are great, and therapy is usually excellent.

HOW DO I TRACK MY RECOVERY?

As I discussed in Chapter 3, the nervous system is connected to every other system in the human body. The muscles, the lymphatic system, the digestive system, the eyes and the other sense organs are all hard-wired to the brain. Athletes can take advantage of this connectivity to monitor their recovery status in various situations—for example, when travelling across time zones or starting an altitude-training camp. But you don't have to be an athlete to use these tools. Anyone who wants to monitor their own responses to stress or training can use the connection between the nervous system and the body to determine whether they're adapting positively or negatively to their environment. This monitoring works because the nervous system detects stress in the body and then sends these signals to the brain. The brain then activates either the parasympathetic nervous system via the vagus nerve, or the sympathetic nervous system via the sympathetic ganglia. If the body is recovering nicely and is in a rested/adaptation condition, then the parasympathetic system dominates and the vagus nerve will slow the heartbeat. Alternatively, if signals are being sent back to the brain indicating that the body is under-recovered, stressed or even trying to fight an infection, then the sympathetic ganglia will increase their activity and the heart rate will increase.

Heart rate can be measured easily with little or no equipment. A simple heart-rate monitor works really well, or you can just take your pulse. We use two test options to monitor an elite athlete's nervous system status and, hence, recovery and regeneration status. These techniques can also predict illness several days before symptoms become visible. So if you do monitor consistently over time, you can detect patterns, and if your heart-rate response is increased, then you can take action—such as choosing an easy workout instead of an interval session—to prevent getting sick. The first test is a simple measurement of your resting heart rate; the second is a more advanced measurement called the Rusko test.

Test Option 1: Measure Resting Heart Rate

This test option is the easiest, lowest-cost and possibly most effective tool you can use to track your recovery status. Simply take your pulse (as described in Chapter 1) for 60 seconds first thing in the morning. Make sure you do this as soon as you wake up and while still lying in bed; even sitting up will increase your heart rate. If you take this measurement every morning, you should notice a relatively constant resting heart rate. Generally speaking, the heart rate of an elite endurance athlete is usually in the 35 to 45 beats per minute range. Relatively healthy active people should have about 55 to 65 beats per minute. If your resting heart rate is over 70, then you should seriously consider increasing your regular physical activity level and starting a stress-management program. Higher-resting heart rates are associated with a greater risk of cardiovascular disease and increased rates of mortality.

Once you have collected some data continually over a few weeks (or a couple of months if you are female—see next paragraph), then you will notice that your resting heart rate changes slightly from day to day. If there's increased stress in your life, or if you had a particularly hard workout the day before, your resting heart rate will likely be higher. If you are doing a training program, as your cardiovascular fitness improves, your resting heart rate will gradually decrease. This decrease in heart rate is a good thing because it shows that the parasympathetic system is starting to gain dominance; your body is letting you know that it is adapting positively to the exercise stimulus.

Women who are interested in using this tool should be aware that their resting heart rate changes depending on what phase of the menstrual cycle is dominant, so monitoring should be done monthly.

Test Option 2: The Rusko Test

This test is the more advanced option. I have people use this test only on a weekly basis, or every day for a short period of time. The reason is that it's much more time intensive (it takes about 10 minutes vs. 1 minute for the resting HR test) and requires using a heart-rate monitor, with a post-analysis of some data. The test was designed by Finnish physiologist Dr. Heikki Rusko, the physiologist for many of the Nordic cross-country skiers who dominated the sport for years. The test works on the same principles as the resting heart-rate test, but also adds in a light cardiovascular stress to trigger your baroreceptors. The baroreceptors, located in the carotid arteries, are sensitive to changes in systemic blood pressure. They activate or relax the smooth muscle tissue controlling the tension in the walls of your blood vessels to regulate blood distribution around the body and ensure that your brain gets the blood flow it needs.

For the Rusko test, you lie down for a period of time so that blood flow is distributed evenly throughout the body and you're as relaxed as possible. Then you stand up quickly. This action forces blood flow into the legs as a result of the pull of gravity, and blood pressure falls. This effect is called orthostatic hypotension and can cause dizziness due to a lack of blood flow to the brain. It is extremely dangerous. It is the same thing that occurs when quickly getting out of a hot tub. To counteract the fall in the brain's blood flow, the fall in blood pressure activates the baroreceptors, signalling the sympathetic nervous system to increase heart rate and contract the leg vasculature to drive blood into the upper body and keep the brain supplied with oxygen. So we see an increase in heart rate upon standing that gradually calms down over a few minutes.

The resting heart rate is quite constant. About 150 seconds into the test, the individual stands up, and the heart rate spikes by almost 40 beats per minute. It then settles down to a new baseline of about 70 beats per minute. If you perform this test on multiple days you can see the impact that stressors such as travel, workouts, or other events can have on the body. Check out the data on the graph below from an athlete who attended an altitude-training camp.

As you can see in the graph, when the athlete is at altitude on Day 1 after travel, the heart-rate response after standing is quite high and does not fall back to a new, lower baseline. Then gradually, as the athlete adapts on days 3 through 5, the heart-rate response returns to normal; in fact, there may even have been some positive adaptation to better than pre-training camp values.

TRAIN WHEN THE BODY IS READY

In the past, coaches would plan training sessions and the athletes would train according to plan no matter what happened or how they felt. More recently, coaches have started to take the athletes' training status into account in the day-to-day management of the training plan. For example, if the coach had planned a speed-training session (which requires intensity and will put the nervous system under stress) and the athletes look sluggish and tired during warm-up, the coach might change the plan immediately. Knowing that an intensity session might not work that day, the coach could change the plan and do a lighter aerobic or technique session and then return to speed work at the following session. This guarantees quality training when the athlete is capable of performing at 100%. It is another example of the aggregate of 1% gains principle that I recommend to achieve world-class health and performance. Evaluate how you are feeling physically and mentally and manage your exercise and nutrition accordingly. If you feel energetic after your warm-up, then go for a high-intensity training session if that is what you had planned. If at the end of your warm-up you still feel tired or have low energy, then do a lighter workout. This will speed your recovery, reduce your stress levels and ultimately increase your energy.

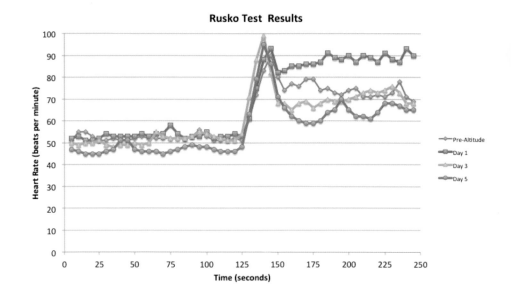

Rusko Test Results

Here are the instructions for the Rusko test:

Before Test

► Set your heart rate–monitoring watch to record your heart rate every 5 seconds.

► Before sleeping, ensure your heart-rate (HR) strap and watch are placed beside your bed, within your grasp while lying on your bed.

Test

► Place the HR strap around your chest when you wake up first thing in the morning. Avoid getting up out of bed while putting on the HR strap.

► Lie on your back for 1 minute after placing the HR strap on your body.

► After 1 minute has passed, start recording your HR.

► Lie still on your back for 3 minutes.

► After the 3 minutes, stand up quickly.

► Stay standing for an additional 2 minutes.

► After the final 2 minutes are complete, stop recording your HR.

► Download the test through the appropriate software.

► Save the text file, and plot the heart rate vs. time data in a spreadsheet to see your results or download our analysis file from my website (www.drgrewells.com and search for Rusko Test).

CONCLUSION

Recovery and regeneration are crucial factors for determining who will be the champions. Those who are committed to taking care of themselves in this way will perform better, more often. This process of care leads to optimal responses physiologically and psychologically. And the best thing about all this information is that anyone can apply these techniques to improve their performance, regardless of the discipline. Try them out for yourself and see what works for you.

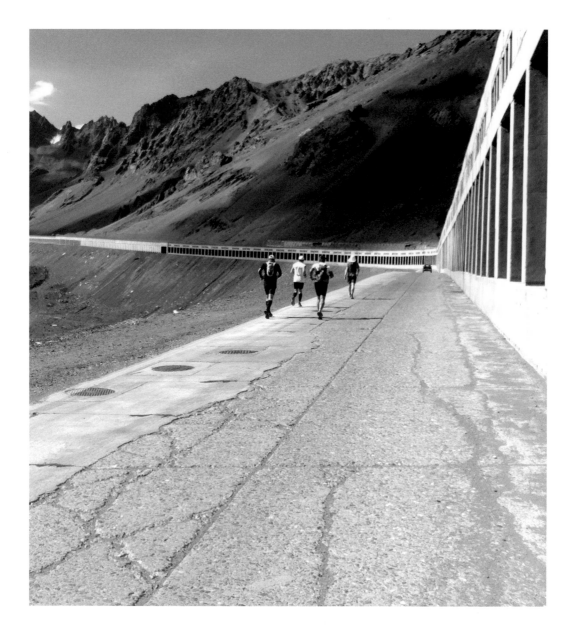

PUTTING IT ALL TOGETHER

THE HUMANETICS™ *APPROACH TO BUILDING A WORLD-CLASS LIFE*

7

To help you set up a physical training plan to achieve the aggregate of 1% gains (as explained in the Introduction) and be able to perform on demand, I'm going to present what I call my "*Humanetics* training model." It's based on scientific discoveries and discussions I've had with some of the world's best coaches. This model is now being used by world-class athletes to deal with the new realities of international competition. I believe that it is also a great model for many people who are interested in improving their general fitness. *Humanetics* is a term that Ray Zahab and I coined to describe the process of applying scientific research to enhance training, performance and health. Ultimately, that is what this book is all about. It is the focus of this chapter, where we will pull all our knowledge about training together to give you a practical plan you can use.

In the 1970s, 1980s and through some of the 1990s, the expectation was that international-level athletes had to peak only once, maybe twice, per year. This expectation led to a popular concept called periodization, where athletes would engage primarily in one form of training (such as endurance training) before moving on to the next type (such as strength development). This training design led to improvements, but problems began to emerge and be noticed by both coaches and scientists. Periodization involves the creation of new proteins because of the effect of training on the DNA. If athletes engage in only one type of training, then only proteins related to that type of exercise are created. For example, if you endurance train, then your body creates new mitochondria and aerobic enzymes. Unfortunately, your body does not maintain structures it does not use. So if you stop that endurance training, the stimulus to create and maintain those aerobic endurance mitochondria and enzymes is decreased, and the gains made through that hard training are lost. Therefore, athletes were faced with trying to maintain gains in one area while developing new capacities in another. Eventually, this dilemma led to the concurrent training model used by many elite athletes and coaches today. This is a model where all energy systems and physical characteristics that are important for achieving the desired end performance are trained concurrently, throughout the season.

Simply put, concurrent training targets all energy systems (high-energy phosphate, anaerobic, and aerobic) as well as strength and power training at the same time. Almost every sport has more than just a single physiological component—except at the extremes. For example, weightlifting is very focused on strength, and the 100-metre dash is almost all high-energy phosphate metabolism. At the other end of the extreme is marathon running, which is almost all aerobic. But for many athletes who train for sports between these extremes, as well as for members of the general population who are interested in building overall health and fitness, concurrent training is the way to go. The benefit of targeting all energy systems and some strength and power training at the same time is that you never lose fitness in any area. Because concurrent training is more complex, and there are only so many hours in a week to train, it results in a slower rate of progress. But it provides long-term improvement and a more comprehensive overall level of fitness and health.

Concurrent training has an added benefit. The new reality in sports at the elite level is that athletes now have to perform at a very high level throughout a longer competitive season. They are required to peak more than once, often as many as 10 to 20 times throughout the year. Competitive resilience is therefore critical now because athletes have to perform on the World Cup circuit, at national championships and at world championships. For example, in 2010 to 2011, national swim teams competed in Delhi for the Commonwealth Games in September, in Dubai at the world short course (25-metre pool) championships in December, at the respective national team trials in April, in Europe at the World Cup events in May and June, and then at the world championships in July. So concurrent training allows athletes to adjust the intensity and volume of their training within a consistent training plan that's only one or two weeks long. This ability permits athletes flexibility on a monthly basis, depending on the competition or training demands they're faced with.

Concurrent training is the perfect model for the general population as well. Throughout the year, we're all faced with exactly the same performance or life demands that athletes face. For example, if we follow a concurrent training model, we can decrease our training while on vacation, or increase our training after holidays to get back into shape after too many cocktail parties. And if we have a light workweek, we can increase our training to take advantage of lower total life stress. Conversely, we can shift our training into more of a recovery focus if personal life or work becomes extremely stressful.

Concurrent training helps keep athletes trained in all aspects of their performance so they are able to compete at an international level more often than previously thought possible. It is also the key to helping average people stay healthy, perform at a high level and manage their life stresses. Furthermore, having a constant change in exercise stimulus is more interesting and fun than slogging away endlessly at only one aspect of your fitness program.

There is one major challenge with concurrent training, however. When we exercise, chemical inductors—those physiological by-products of exercise that signal DNA to produce proteins and structures, helping us adapt to the training stress—are created. This adaptation benefits the body and we get stronger, faster or fitter. But these chemical inductors have an interesting property. They also block adaptation in exercise capacities opposed to the type of exercise being performed. This phenomenon is called "interference effects,"[82] and it occurs when inductors blunt improvements in other, unrelated areas.[83] For example, marathoners tend to develop lean muscles that are full of mitochondria, whereas weightlifters have big, thick muscles that are full of actin and myosin contractile proteins. When we do endurance exercise, the activity of the enzyme AMP kinase increases. Although this increase improves mitochondrial metabolism, it nevertheless dampens improvements in the muscles' strength apparatus. Conversely, when we strength train (by lifting weights, for example), a molecule called mTOR is produced. mTOR is involved in the signalling process that helps muscles adapt to become stronger, but it also slows adaptation in the mitochondria. Scientists are not sure how long interference effects last, but our best guess is about 12 to 24 hours. So this timing leads to a critical point for anyone interested in training: It is essential to do the most important aspect of your training before you do anything else. For example, if today is an aerobic day, make sure that you do the main aerobic-training set as early in the practice as possible. If sprinting is the focus, be sure to do this early in the practice, and do any other physiological work later. To avoid interference effects and to

THE BEST TIME OF DAY TO EXERCISE

Ultimately, the best time of day to exercise is when you can fit it into your schedule consistently. Mornings are great because there are fewer chances that the events of the day will derail your workout plans. Training in the afternoon, however, may be better from a performance perspective. We all have circadian rhythms that adjust our metabolism throughout the day, the month and maybe even the year. But on a daily basis, our body temperature changes, and for most of us it is highest in the afternoon. Higher body temperatures are associated with improved muscle performance. So training in the afternoon is a good option for you if you can be consistent.

plan an effective training program, I'll show you the training zones that I use to help me analyze exercise and sport performance.

THE SEVEN KEY TRAINING ZONES

I build my training plans based on seven training zones that cover the ranges of energy systems from ATP (adenosine triphosphate) right through to purely aerobic. I decided to define the training zones to reflect the well-established power–duration relationship that exists for humans (and most other animals as well).[84] The power-duration relationship and the training zones are shown in the graph on page 193.

The training zones I have defined in the graph are summarized over the next few pages. These zones are: (1) the aerobic-base zone, (2) the Aerobic-threshold-zone, (3) the aerobic-power-zone, (4) the anaerobic-tolerance zone, (5) the anaerobic-power-zone, (6) the high-energy phosphate capacity zone and (7) the power zone.

Aerobic-Base-Zone Training

This type of training is the foundation for most people, even elite athletes. It is used to improve the aerobic and cardiovascular system and to build a good base level of fitness. More specifically, aerobic-base-zone training is used for developing an aerobic fitness foundation and improving cardiovascular health and endurance. If you are new to fitness training, this is where you need to spend the most time over the first few months.

Aerobic-base training involves performing low-intensity exercise typically at 50 to 65% of your maximum heart rate. This can be done for longer periods—for example, a 40-minute run or bike at a constant, even intensity with minimal or no rest. When doing aerobic-zone training, you should be able to hear yourself breathe but still be able to carry on a conversation. You should feel like you're putting in some exercise effort, but at an intensity that you could sustain for an extended period relatively comfortably.

Aerobic-base sessions can last from 15 minutes if you're just starting out to more than 3 hours if you're an endurance athlete. For most of us, a 45- to

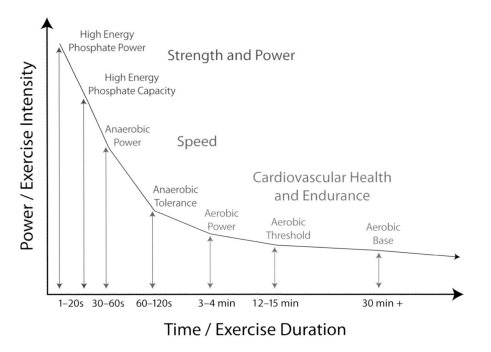

Y-axis: Power / Exercise Intensity

X-axis: Time / Exercise Duration

Chart labels:
- High Energy Phosphate Power
- Strength and Power
- High Energy Phosphate Capacity
- Anaerobic Power
- Speed
- Cardiovascular Health and Endurance
- Anaerobic Tolerance
- Aerobic Power
- Aerobic Threshold
- Aerobic Base

X-axis intervals: 1–20s 30–60s 60–120s 3–4 min 12–15 min 30 min +

60-minute easy run or bike is what aerobic-base training is all about. Here's how a workout might look.

Activation

Perform light activation movements such as walking lunges, squats, trunk rotations or arm circles for 5 minutes. Once you've finished loosening up, you can begin your main workout.

Main set

Perform some cardiovascular exercise in your aerobic-base zone (50–65% HR_{max}). Walking, swimming, rowing, cycling, jogging, elliptical, flow yoga, etc., would all qualify. Just keep your HR constant for the whole workout and minimize breaks between exercises. The main set can last from 15 minutes to several hours.

Active recovery

Perform some very light cardiovascular exercise such as walking for 5 minutes. Finish your workout with some stretching. Hold stretches for at least 15 seconds. Calves, quadriceps, hamstrings, glutes, chest, back and neck are muscle areas you can work on stretching.

Aerobic-threshold-zone training is challenging and requires a reasonably strong effort. Threshold-zone training is important for athletes who have already established a good level of aerobic base conditioning and for people who are looking for a tougher workout that will increase their fitness rapidly. If you are trying this type of workout for the first time, make sure that you're comfortable with aerobic-base-zone training before beginning.

Aerobic-threshold training involves pushing the body to work for extended periods at or near where it starts to accumulate some lactic acid. Some people refer to this level of intensity as the anaerobic threshold, the maximal-lactic steady state or even the critical-power state, among other names. Typically, aerobic-threshold intervals are performed at 65 to 80% of your maximum heart rate. Your breathing will be laboured. As a result of the increased intensity, aerobic-threshold training often involves breaking up the exercise into intervals. Intervals are shorter exercise blocks (usually a few minutes long) that are separated by a rest period; for example, 45 seconds at 50% effort, 45 seconds at 65 to 80% effort, repeated a number of times. The exercise duration can be increased from 45 seconds up to 10 minutes or even longer as your fitness improves, and the rest can also be adjusted to make the training more difficult (less rest) or easier (more rest). The total duration of the interval-training set can be adjusted from just a few minutes when starting out to up to 60 minutes for highly trained athletes. Make sure you work with a trainer or fitness professional to design the interval-training sessions and to incorporate the sessions into your overall fitness program.

Here is an example.

Activation

Perform light activation movements such as walking lunges, squats, trunk rotations or arm circles for 5 minutes. Then perform 30 seconds at 40% HR_{max}, followed by 30 seconds at 65% HR_{max}. Repeat 5 times. Take 2 minutes of easy exercise, then begin your main set.

Main set

Alternate periods of high-intensity exercise with active recovery.

Example   1:15 × 1 minute at 75% HR_{max} alternated with 1 minute at 50% HR_{max}. Set time: 30 minutes

Example   *2:5 × 3 minutes at 70% HR$_{max}$ alternated with 90 seconds at 50% HR$_{max}$.*
                    Set time: 22.5 minutes

Example   *3:4 × 6 minutes at 65% HR$_{max}$ alternated with 2 minutes at 50% HR$_{max}$.*
                    Set time: 32 minutes

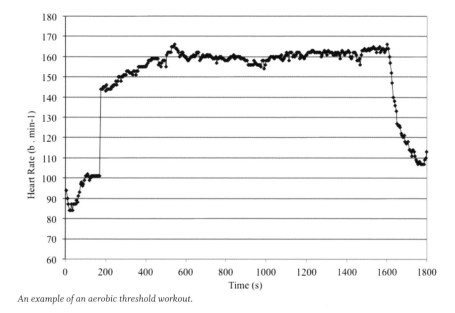

An example of an aerobic threshold workout.

Training in the aerobic-threshold zone will increase your ability to exercise at a relatively high intensity for an extended period. On page 197 is an example of a heart-rate profile from an athlete who performed an approximately 20-minute effort at his aerobic threshold.

Active recovery
Perform some very light cardiovascular exercise for 5 to 10 minutes. Finish with some stretching. Hold stretches at least 15 seconds.

Aerobic-Power-Zone Training
Aerobic-power-zone training is highly challenging. This type of training formed the foundation of the Australian swimming team's success for many years. It's also been used by people such as Lance Armstrong in other sports to build the capacity of the cardiovascular and the aerobic energy

systems with the ultimate objective of increasing endurance capacity. When someone performs aerobic-power-zone training, the cardiovascular and aerobic energy systems are maximally activated, meaning that the heart, lungs, blood and mitochondria in the muscle are all working near or at their maximum. Because the body is working so hard there is also significant activation of the anaerobic system, which means that sugars are being broken down for energy and there's going to be some accumulation of lactic acid in the muscle and blood. This type of training is very, very tough. But it also pays huge dividends in the way it stimulates the body to adapt. This zone is extremely effective for building endurance and cardiovascular fitness.

More specifically, during aerobic-power-training sets, heart rates are often in excess of 80% of maximum and lactate levels can reach 6 to 8 mmol/L. Intervals can last from 45 seconds to several minutes. The rest in between can be from 30 seconds to several minutes. The total time the aerobic-power intervals add up to should not exceed more than a few minutes for people new to this type of training. Even the elite athletes who use this training rarely exceed 40 minutes of total work.

Here is an example.

Activation

Perform light activation movements such as walking lunges, squats, trunk rotations or arm circles for 5 minutes. Then perform 30 seconds at 40% HR_{max}, followed by 30 seconds at 65% HR_{max}. Repeat 10 times. Take 2 minutes of easy exercise. You can then begin your main set.

Main set

Alternate between periods of very high intensity exercise with active recovery. Here is a classic aerobic power set for elite endurance athletes:

> 20×1 minute at 80 to 90% of HR_{max} alternating with
> 30 seconds of passive rest

An introductory version of this set may simply be shorter and have some active recovery between the intense intervals:

> 5×45 seconds at 80% of HR_{max} alternating with
> 45 seconds of light activity at 50% HR_{max}

Modifications can be made by increasing the length of the intervals. I don't like going any longer than 4 minutes of sustained effort for aerobic power training, so here is an example of how far you may someday be able to go with this type of training set:

> 6×4 minutes at 80 to 90% of HR_{max} alternating with
> 1 to 2 minutes of light activity at 50% HR_{max}

In a particularly brutal practice leading into the 2004 Olympics, an athlete I was working with did a set of 15×4 minutes with a 2-minute rest interval. The graph below shows what the heart rate curve looked like.

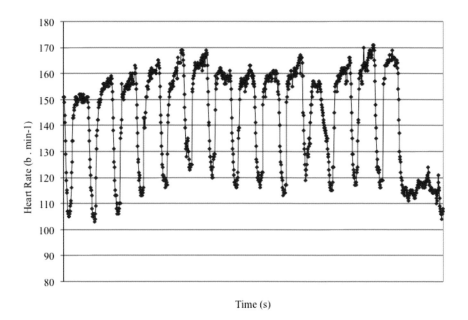

Interval training involves periods of hard work alternating with periods of rest.

The benefits of interval training are due to the fact that the hard part of the training is at a high rather than a constant level. Researchers believe that interval training is the best way to improve cardiovascular fitness and endurance. Even though parts of the workout are at a lower intensity, the body is working hard to recover and remove waste products created by the high-intensity sections. So even the low-intensity parts are challenging to the muscles and the blood.

When you are learning to move into the aerobic-power zone, you can also do "descending" sets. In this case, you alternate an interval that becomes progressively more challenging with a recovery interval that's done at a constant moderate intensity. These sets would look like this:

1×2 minutes at 55% HR$_{max}$ alternating with
1 minute active recovery at 50% HR$_{max}$

1×2 minutes at 60% HR$_{max}$ alternating with
1 minute active recovery at 50% HR$_{max}$

1×2 minutes at 65% HR$_{max}$ alternating with
1 minute active recovery at 50% HR$_{max}$

1×2 minutes at 70% HR$_{max}$ alternating with
1 minute active recovery at 50% HR$_{max}$

1×2 minutes at 75% HR$_{max}$ alternating with
1 minute active recovery at 50% HR$_{max}$

1×2 minutes at 80% HR$_{max}$ alternating with
1 minute active recovery at 50% HR$_{max}$

1×2 minutes at 85% HR$_{max}$ alternating with
1 minute active recovery at 50% HR$_{max}$

This is a great way of warming the body up and learning what it feels like to work in the aerobic-power zone.

Active recovery
Always finish an aerobic-power set with some very light cardiovascular exercise for 5 to 10 minutes. End with some stretching. Hold stretches at least 15 seconds.

Warning. Aerobic-power-zone training is highly challenging and demanding. Consult your physician before starting this type of training. I would recommend a minimum of 6 months of consistent training in the aerobic-base zone and the Aerobic-threshold-zone before even attempting a workout in the aerobic-power zone. Stop exercising and consult your doctor immediately if you experience any pain or dizziness.

Anaerobic-Tolerance-Zone Training

In this training zone, the objective is to build up the body's ability to produce energy through the aerobic system and tolerate the fatigue-inducing effects of the "acid" component of lactic acid. Training in the anaerobic zone is very tough because it usually involves exercising at a high enough intensity that the body has to break down sugars using the anaerobic system inside muscle. This process causes a great deal of fatigue, which can be interpreted as "pain" or muscle discomfort. Also, when lactic acid is produced, the increased levels of hydrogen ions and carbon dioxide that accumulate activate the breathing control centres of the body and you feel that we have to breathe very hard and that you can't catch your breath. In general, this feeling is very uncomfortable. On the benefits side, anaerobic training is highly effective because, even when you're recovering from an anaerobic effort, your aerobic system is working to help you out. So it's a very efficient use of your time. There is also growing evidence that training in this zone (and in the anaerobic-power zone, described next) is very good for your brain's health and for preventing chronic disease in a variety of organ systems.

Anaerobic training can also be lots of fun. Think sprint and rest, sprint and rest. Interestingly, this is the way children play. Just watch them in the park. They'll have bursts of energy and then will walk around for a while. People think of hockey, basketball, soccer and other team sports as lots of fun—and they are. But most of these sports involve alternating periods of high-intensity exercise with lower-intensity periods of recovery.

When you do anaerobic training, monitoring your heart rate is not appropriate because you're not concerned about oxygen delivery or use. You're interested in working hard enough to produce lactic acid. Fortunately, at least for monitoring purposes, breathing and the anaerobic system are closely linked. Using Dr. Robert Goode's Talk Test (described in Chapter 1), you want to work hard enough that you can't carry on a conversation. You should be experiencing some muscle burning or heaviness, and you will likely feel some significant muscle fatigue. If you were to rank your exercise intensity from 1 to 20, with 1 being sitting on the couch and 20 being the hardest sprint you've ever done in your life, anaerobic exercise needs to be in the 14 to 20 range. If you have access to a blood-lactate analyzer, the anaerobic-tolerance zone is from 5 to 8 mmol/L.

HOW TO COMBINE MUSCLE AND AEROBIC TRAINING

So far I've described how to do aerobic-base, threshold and power training. Mostly I've referred to time intervals for the exercise efforts and recovery pieces of the workout that are needed to build the training session. You can do these workouts swimming, running, cycling, rowing or using gym equipment such as stair climbers. But you can also do these workouts to target your muscle strength and endurance development by lifting weights in the gym.

As I discussed in Chapter 2, anyone can train to increase muscle endurance (low weight, high repetitions), muscle strength (heavy weight, 8 to 12 repetitions) and muscle power (low–medium weight, high-velocity movement, low repetitions).

You can build muscle training into your aerobic workouts as well. Here are some examples of how to do this.

Aerobic-base muscle-endurance training

To do this type of training in the gym, you can use what is often called circuit training. Pick as many exercises as you want and then perform them in sequence with minimal rest. You can keep the weights light so that your heart rate stays constantly elevated, but in the right zone. For example, you could do (1) push-ups, (2) squats, (3) lunges, (4) back arches, (5) lateral pull-downs, (6) rowing, (7) abdominal crunches and (8) step-ups. You could do each exercise for 45 seconds and then take 15 seconds to change stations. Then just work your way around the circuit 1 to 3 times to create your aerobic training session. Just remember to warm up and do active recovery following the session. Wear a heart-rate monitor or check your pulse periodically to make sure you are in the 50 to 65% of your maximum zone.

Aerobic-threshold muscle-endurance training

To work your aerobic-threshold in the gym using weights or machines, you simply have to increase the intensity of the work that you're doing by increasing the weight slightly and/or increasing the tempo of the exercises that you're performing. Circuits work great for this as well, and once again it is a good idea to monitor your heart rate to make sure you are in the target zone of 65 to 80% of your maximum. Another great way to create longer intervals that challenge the body is to do something called "supersets." In this case, you can alternate two different exercises that target different muscle groups; for example, push-ups for the upper body and squats for the lower body. Then simply cycle back and forth between the exercises to hit your target heart-rate zone and desired interval length. Recovery between supersets can be passive (e.g., just relaxing; not recommended) or active (e.g., riding a stationary bike or walking). Here's an example of an aerobic-threshold superset workout. (Remember to warm up and do active recovery following the session.)

Superset 1

EXERCISE	TARGET AREA	REPETITIONS	REST INTERVAL
Push-ups	Upper body	20	None
Squats	Lower body	20	None

Alternate push-ups and squats 3 times. Allow 2 minutes of active recovery following the superset before moving on to superset 2.

Superset 2

EXERCISE	TARGET AREA	REPETITIONS	REST INTERVAL
Crunches on stability ball	Abdominals	20	None
Lunges	Lower body	20	None

Alternate crunches and lunges 3 times. Allow 2 minutes of active recovery following the superset before moving on to superset 3. Alternating muscle groups with minimal rest between sets creates significant cardiovascular stress and trains specific muscle groups concurrently.

Superset 3

EXERCISE	TARGET AREA	REPETITIONS	REST INTERVAL
Push-ups	Upper body	15	60 seconds skipping
Squats	Lower body	15	60 seconds skipping
Crunches on stability ball	Abdominals	15	60 seconds skipping
Lunges	Lower body	15	60 seconds skipping

Allow 4 minutes of active recovery at 50% of maximum heart rate.

The above cycle may be repeated (or the structure repeated with different exercises). Remember, if you are starting out it is best to get used to the aerobic-base and threshold-type workouts before attempting the more intense aerobic power sessions.

Aerobic-power muscle-endurance training

In this case, we are looking to train the cardiovascular system and the muscle endurance at or near the limit of the cardiovascular and aerobic systems' capacity. Just as I've noted in the aerobic-base and the threshold muscle-endurance explanations, this training is possible to achieve in the gym. The same principles can be applied: Make sure to warm up well before the exercises, monitor your heart rate and do active recovery after the session. Then create a circuit or superset session of sufficient intensity to push the cardiovascular system into the Aerobic-power-zone. Increasing intensity can be accomplished by increasing the weight or the tempo of the exercises as described in Chapter 2. You can also decrease the rest and recovery allowed between exercises. A great way to do this is to add skipping as "recovery" between exercises—an activity that keeps the exercise stress constant, yet changes muscle groups just enough to allow some recovery so you can move on to the next exercise and keep the training session progressing.

The key to the anaerobic-tolerance zone is to produce some lactic acid by activating the anaerobic glycolytic system through high-intensity exercise and then keep the lactic acid levels elevated for a period of time. Once again, alternating exercise and recovery works very well. The rest duration should be sufficient to keep the exercise intensity high. Typically, a 1:3 work:rest ratio is ideal because it takes 2 or 3 minutes for lactic acid to be transported from the muscle into the blood. The result is that the subsequent interval begins when there's lactic acid in both the muscle and the blood; hence, the term "anaerobic tolerance." I strongly recommend some low-intensity active recovery between repetitions because this will help clear the lactic acid that has been produced and improve the quality of the high-intensity intervals. Here's an example of how to structure an anaerobic-tolerance zone workout:

Activation

Perform light activation movements such as walking lunges, squats, trunk rotations or arm circles for five minutes. For some examples of activation movements, check out Appendix 1. Follow this routine with an aerobic warm-up including at least 10 minutes of moderate-intensity cardiovascular activity. Once you've finished loosening up you can begin your main workout.

Main set

Repetitions	Interval duration	Intensity	Rest interval
4–30	30–60 seconds	maximum	90 seconds–3 minutes (1 : 3 work : rest)

Moderate-intensity exercise for 10 minutes can be added at any time to clear the waste products from the muscles.

Active recovery

Perform some very light cardiovascular exercise such as walking or cycling for at least 15 minutes. Finish your workout with some stretching. Hold stretches for at least 15 seconds.

Anaerobic-Power-Zone Training

Anaerobic-power-zone training takes the anaerobic-tolerance zone just a bit farther. The objective in the anaerobic-power-zone is to train the muscles and the anaerobic glycolytic–energy system to produce energy as quickly as possible when breaking down sugars and carbohydrates. The outcome of this is very high levels of lactic acid in the muscle and blood, but also very high muscle-power outputs. This is the key training zone for improving speed that lasts longer than 20 seconds.

Because anaerobic-power-zone training results in the production of very high levels of lactic acid, it's quite uncomfortable. Lactate levels should approach maximum, which often means between 8 and 20 mmol/L, depending on the individual. On our perceived-effort scale, the goal is to try to reach an intensity between 18 and 20. Working in this zone builds speed and the ability to exercise at higher intensities across a range of sports, even in endurance events (e.g., it helps you build the capacity to run up hills in running races). To do this type of training properly, lots of rest is required (at least a 1:6 work:rest ratio). Low-intensity active recovery between repetitions is recommended. Also, because the carbohydrate energy stores in the body are limited, the total high-intensity work should be limited to 6 to 8 minutes. Always follow this type of exercise training with carbohydrate snacks and meals to help replenish muscle-glycogen stores and speed recovery.

An aerobic-power-zone workout is usually a challenging cardiovascular workout that involves high-intensity efforts that are repeated a number of times. Examples include interval training, running hills or other types of activities that drive heart rate and oxygen demand to very high levels. Here's an example of how to structure an anaerobic-power-zone workout:

Activation
Perform light activation movements such as walking lunges, squats, trunk rotations or arm circles for 5 minutes. Follow this routine with an aerobic warm-up including at least 10 minutes of moderate-intensity cardiovascular activity. Once you've finished warming up, you can begin your main workout.

Main set:

Repetitions	Interval duration	Intensity	Rest interval
6	60 seconds	maximum	6 minutes (1 : 6 work : rest)

Or

Repetitions	Interval duration	Intensity	Rest interval
3	120 seconds	maximum	12 minutes (1 : 6 work : rest)

Active recovery should be included during the rest interval between high-intensity efforts.

Active recovery

Perform some very light cardiovascular exercise such as walking or cycling for at least 15 minutes. Finish your workout with some stretching. Hold stretches for at least 15 seconds.

High-Energy Phosphate Capacity and Power-Zone Training

High-energy phosphates (HEPs) are the sources of energy for immediate high-intensity exercise. We have about 10 seconds of an energy source called adenosine triphosphate (ATP) and about 20 seconds' worth of energy from phosphocreatine (PCr). Breaking down ATP and PCr in the muscle releases huge amounts of energy very quickly, and there are no waste products that directly cause fatigue. So these energy sources are great for short bursts of high-intensity exercise.

If we do this type of exercise—short bursts of high-intensity activities—we can increase the amount of ATP and PCr in our muscles, and we can also increase the number and concentration of enzymes that break down these structures. So we end up with more stored energy and we can break it down faster. The outcome is that we can run faster, jump higher and throw farther as well as improve our agility and other athletic abilities. Sports that rely on this system include volleyball (indoor and outdoor), badminton, squash and tennis, as well as gymnastics and the shorter events in track and field.

To train in this zone, the intervals must be short. Exercise bouts of less than 10 seconds target the high-energy phosphate system and specifically ATP breakdown. We call this HEP power training. If we do high-intensity exercise that lasts a bit longer (about 15 to 20 seconds), it stresses both ATP and PCR stores and enzymes. We call this HEP-capacity training. Successful training in this zone is done at very high intensities and is lots of fun, but demands concentration and effort. And rest is critical. Unlike in anaerobic training, resting between HEP intervals needs to be very passive. Many track athletes lie down and barely move between training intervals. It usually takes about 3 minutes for replenishment of the high-energy phosphate stores, so I recommend taking at least that much rest time between exercise bouts. It is important to note that, because the intensity of exercise is very high, so is the risk of injury. So be careful, and use perfect technique at all times. This is one area where having a professional trainer or coach is critical.

Exercises or intervals that are executed to train HEP capacity and power can be sport-specific—running sprints or tennis serves are examples. Alternatively, you can train to improve muscle function in these zones by doing muscle strength and power exercises in the gym. Just stick to the short work intervals and long 3-minute rest intervals to make sure you are working in the right training zone.

Now that we have defined training zones, the next step is to build a week training plan.

THE BASIC WEEK PLAN

I have taken all the information from the earlier chapters of this book into account and built a single-week training plan that's comprehensive and highly effective and that avoids interference effects. In general, I recommend that all people work toward having at least 6 hours a week of physical activity. Although this requirement may seem like quite a lot of exercise, most of the research I have read supports 6 hours as the threshold volume of activity needed to improve fitness, prevent chronic disease and improve brain function and capacity. Dr. John Ratey has written a brilliant book on the effects of exercise on the brain called *Spark*. He also subscribes to the 6 hours per week threshold, although his focus is on using exercise for improving mental skills such as concentration and problem-solving, as well as alleviating such clinical conditions as depression, anxiety and dementia. The concurrent training model I propose here targets not only the brain, but also all the body systems described in this book, including the heart, lungs, blood and muscle, as well as the endocrine and nervous systems.

For those who are just starting to incorporate exercise into their lives, 6 hours may be too much. Feel free to decrease the duration of each session when you are starting out, but try to stick to the exercise modalities that I've recommended. Even as little as 15 minutes of exercise has been shown to increase blood markers for the metabolites that process fats, sugars and amino acids by 70% in people who have low levels of fitness. As you increase your fitness you can increase the duration and intensity of each session. But again, try to stick to the week plan structure outlined in the text that follows. I'm going to lead you through the physiology and rationale for the concurrent week plan beginning with the foundation of exercise performance and health—cardiovascular exercise.

As I discussed in Chapter 1, cardiovascular exercise has powerful positive effects on almost every system in the human body. It improves exercise capacity, sharpens brain skills such as problem-solving and concentration and prevents chronic disease. Therefore, this form of exercise is the foundation of the concurrent training model. I recommend people start their week with some light cardiovascular exercise on Monday mornings. This beginning helps people get into the routine of the week and prepares the brain for the tasks to be performed to get the week started. Let's add this feature to the training plan. I've noted that Monday morning is to be done at a low intensity or in the aerobic-base-training zone (at 50 to 65% of your maximum heart rate). The time of the session can be 15 to 90 minutes, depending on your fitness level and time commitment. Let's add that session to the week plan.

	SESSION 1 ZONE	EXAMPLE
MONDAY	Aerobic base	Walking, jogging, biking or swimming at low HR
TUESDAY		
WEDNESDAY		
THURSDAY		
FRIDAY		
SATURDAY		
SUNDAY		

The second critical item to add is some cardiovascular training that builds your endurance capacity and stimulates the anaerobic system. This

requirement means you have to exercise in the threshold-training zone and/
or the aerobic-power-training zone. For quick reference, it means you have
to do intervals (e.g., 30 to 90 seconds) at or above your second physiological
threshold, which happens at about 65 to 80% of your maximum heart rate
for the aerobic-threshold workout and 80%+ for the aerobic-power workout.
I prefer to perform these workouts on Tuesdays and Thursdays. Let's add
these to our week plan.

	SESSION 1 ZONE	EXAMPLE
MONDAY	Aerobic base	Walking, jogging, biking or swimming at low HR
TUESDAY	Aerobic threshold	Running or jogging with some sustained efforts
WEDNESDAY		
THURSDAY	Aerobic threshold or power	Exercising with some high-intensity intervals
FRIDAY		
SATURDAY		
SUNDAY		

If you then add some recovery sessions after each hard training session on
Tuesday and Thursday, you have a basic week plan.

	SESSION 1 ZONE	EXAMPLE
MONDAY	Aerobic base	Walking, jogging, biking or swimming at low HR
TUESDAY	Aerobic threshold	Running or jogging with some sustained efforts
WEDNESDAY	Aerobic base	Cycling at a low–moderate heart rate
THURSDAY	Aerobic threshold or power	Running with some hills or intervals
FRIDAY	Aerobic base	Flow yoga
SATURDAY		
SUNDAY		

This is an excellent plan for people in the early stages of exercising for
fitness, although Zone 3 training should be done only after you are very
comfortable with exercising in Zones 1 and 2 and have several months of
background training with a good base level of fitness. That's why I've left
Thursday as aerobic-threshold or power. In the earlier stages of training

and fitness, aerobic-threshold training is more effective, fun and safe than aerobic power. Note that if you add some fun activities on the weekend, you can easily get to the 6 hours per week of recommended exercise.

The next step is to add muscle-resistance training. To learn more about how your muscles respond to strength and power training, review Chapter 2. You need at least two muscle-training sessions per week. These can be muscle endurance, strength or power, depending on your fitness level and overall training goals. For general fitness, I recommend one muscle-endurance session and one muscle strength session per week. Once your fitness level increases or if you are preparing to play sports such as basketball or volleyball, I'd replace the muscle-endurance session with a muscle-power session. If you are looking to improve your body composition and lose some body fat, then I'd suggest doing all your muscle-resistance workouts according to the muscle-strength principles I've outlined.

These resistance workouts can be done in the gym with weights or other apparatus such as stability balls. Afternoons are perfect for this type of work. Let's add these items to the plan.

	SESSION 1 ZONE	EXAMPLE	SESSION 2 ZONE	EXAMPLE
MONDAY	Aerobic base	Walking, jogging, biking or swimming at low HR	Muscle strength	Resistance training in the gym
TUESDAY	Aerobic threshold	Running or jogging with some sustained efforts		
WEDNESDAY	Aerobic base	Cycling at a low-moderate heart rate	Muscle endurance	Circuit training in the gym
THURSDAY	Aerobic threshold or power	Running with some hills or intervals		
FRIDAY	Aerobic base	Flow yoga		
SATURDAY				
SUNDAY				

The final element to add to the plan is, of course, *fun*. I prefer to keep Saturdays for outdoor activities that are of longer duration. You can also keep Saturdays as flexible time to catch up on workouts missed during the week. Also, since most of us don't work on Saturdays, we can participate in activities that don't have a time limit. Longer runs or bike rides are perfect, as are hikes with your family. Any activity works. For individuals training for marathons, triathlons or other sporting events, weekend mornings are the best time to get in longer-volume sessions. I label these sessions as "fun" activity/sport specific to reflect these comments. The week plan now looks like this:

	SESSION 1 ZONE	EXAMPLE	SESSION 2 ZONE	EXAMPLE
MONDAY	Aerobic base	Walking, jogging, biking or swimming at low HR	Muscle strength	Resistance training in the gym
TUESDAY	Aerobic threshold	Running or jogging with some sustained efforts		
WEDNESDAY	Aerobic base	Cycling at a low-moderate heart rate	Muscle endurance	Circuit training in the gym
THURSDAY	Aerobic threshold or power	Running with some hills or intervals		
FRIDAY	Aerobic base	Flow yoga		
SATURDAY	FUN activities	Hiking, playing in the park, etc.	Or sport-specific training	Long run or long training ride
SUNDAY	OFF			

I recommend that you take one day off per week from structured exercise. Going for walks or other types of light physical activity is always okay, but try to give your body and mind a good rest one day a week. This day can be during the week to allow you to focus on work pressures or manage additional family responsibilities.

There is another critical element to add to the week plan. It is something that most people don't consider, but I believe it is the single most important element that ensures your training keeps you healthy and you perform at your best. This critical training element is also guaranteed to help improve your immune system, prevent chronic disease, reduce your stress and speed your regeneration from training. This element is working on your flexibility. To do this, I recommend stretching and yoga or meditation.

Yoga, something I recommend for my athletes and business clients, is a series of exercises designed to develop strength and flexibility while incorporating controlled breathing and mindfulness. It is very powerful and there are many kinds of yoga. Experiment by taking classes from the different schools of yoga until you find one that is right for you. Try to do this once or twice a week, or more if you really enjoy it. Yoga is particularly good for you after a stressful day. You'll discover how your mental stresses manifest themselves in physical tension, and the guided stretching that you do in yoga will help to dissipate the negative physical effects of our busy Western lifestyles. Meditation is another powerful technique for mental relaxation and regeneration. To learn more about this technique, check out a meditation class in your area or read Osho's book, *Meditation: The First and Last Freedom*.

If your body needs some additional help recovering or if you have some physical tension that needs to be addressed, then I strongly recommend massage. I prefer sports massage because it targets tight muscles and helps them to release and recover, but other forms of massage are equally powerful in helping the mind and body to recovery more quickly from exercise training and the stresses of life. Find a great practitioner in your area and see if you can arrange for a weekly, monthly or twice-monthly massage. Often massage schools have excellent therapists available weekly at very low prices. If you have health benefits at work, then see if massage is covered.

I recommend some form of focused recovery, as outlined above, a few times a week. The best times are afternoons or weekends, when you're more likely to need to recover and regenerate. This element helps you recover from the harder training sessions. Spending some time on your physical and mental recovery in the middle of the week helps you arrive at the weekend feeling energetic and healthy. It leads to better exercise training, superior work performance, and increased mental and physical health. Let's add that to our week plan.

	SESSION 1 ZONE	EXAMPLE	SESSION 2 ZONE	EXAMPLE
MONDAY	Aerobic base	Walking, jogging, biking or swimming at low HR	Muscle strength	Resistance training in the gym
TUESDAY	Aerobic threshold	Running or jogging with some sustained efforts	Recovery session*	After-work stretching
WEDNESDAY	Aerobic base	Cycling at a low–moderate heart rate	Muscle endurance	Circuit training in the gym
THURSDAY	Aerobic threshold or power	Running with some hills or intervals	Recovery session*	Massage
FRIDAY	Aerobic base	Flow Yoga		
SATURDAY	Fun activities	Hiking, playing in the park, etc.	Or sport-specific training	Long run or long training ride
SUNDAY	Off			

* A recovery session can be any of the following: yoga, stretching, foam-roller work, massage, meditation or hot/cold contrast baths.

The basic plan I just described is excellent for building and maintaining a base level of fitness. It also works very well for people with busy lives since it allows for recovery after each exercise session and can be adjusted to match your fitness level and personal demands on a weekly basis. Remember, if you are just getting started, then you can do as little as 15 minutes of each of the workouts and experience some benefits. You can also do sessions 1 and 2 on each day back to back if you don't want to do two separate training sessions in one day. Ultimately, I'd recommend that you try to get to 45 minutes per workout and then accumulate 6 hours of total exercise per week. People who are more advanced can still use this program if they increase the workouts to between 60 and 90 minutes, and then gradually increase the total volume and intensity of each workout. It's also important to incorporate recovery into the total plan. So make sure that every fourth training week is a very easy week. A month plan may look something like this:

▶ Week 1. Build the base: 30-minute workouts, low to moderate intensity.
▶ Week 2. Increase capacity: 45-minute workouts, moderate to high intensity.
▶ Week 3. Do hard training: 60-minute workouts, moderate to high intensity.
▶ Week 4. Recover: 30 to 40 minute workouts, low intensity. Emphasis is on evening recovery sessions.

Good luck building your health and performance with the concurrent training plan. Let me know how it goes for you on Twitter (www.twitter.com/drgregwells).

THE ADVANCED WEEK PLAN

The basic plan I have just described is a great way to get started when you're building your fitness, or if you just want to stay in shape and manage your life pressures to maximize your performance and health. But some people who are reaching a higher level of fitness or are training for more advanced events may be interested in a more advanced plan. I've built a week template for athletes in sports that involve multiple energy systems. This plan covers most components of fitness and is great for people looking to build lifelong world-class health and physical capacity. In this plan, nutrition and recovery become critical, because the training load is significantly higher. It's also important to monitor your total stress load so that you don't lose the strength of the immune system and its capacity to keep you healthy.

More advanced training requires adding anaerobic and high-energy phosphate (HEP) workouts. I put anaerobic sessions in on afternoons and add some high-energy phosphate training to the aerobic base workouts on Wednesday and Friday. Allowing at least 24 hours between anaerobic sessions ensures that there is enough time for muscle glycogen to be replaced. The more advanced and comprehensive week plan, which now includes anaerobic and HEP training, looks like this:

	SESSION 1 ZONE	EXAMPLE	SESSION 2 ZONE	EXAMPLE
MONDAY	Aerobic base	Walking, jogging, biking or swimming at low HR	Anaerobic tolerance	Spinning class
TUESDAY	Aerobic Threshold	Running or jogging with some sustained efforts	Muscle strength	Resistance training in the gym
WEDNESDAY	Aerobic base + HEP (jump, throw, sprint, speed)	Cycling at a low-moderate heart rate	Anaerobic power	Running sprints with lots of rest
THURSDAY	Aerobic threshold or power	Running with some hills or intervals	Muscle endurance	Circuit training in the gym
FRIDAY	Aerobic Base + HEP (jump, throw, sprint, speed)	Flow yoga	Recovery session	Light stretching at home
SATURDAY	Fun activities	Hiking, playing in the park, etc.	Or sport-specific training	Long run or long training ride
SUNDAY	Off		Recovery session	Massage

With this plan you can build endurance, strength, power and speed as well as flexibility. There are 10 to 12 workouts per week. As in the basic plan, these workouts can vary in duration from 15 to 120+ minutes per workout. The total volume for the week can therefore range from 6 hours to more than 20 hours, depending on the length of each workout. This much may seem like a lot of training, but I supervise athletes on this plan who train up to 26 hours per week + their recovery sessions. The key to the successful implementation of a training plan like this one is to start very slowly, build very gradually, work in recovery weeks at least once per month, decrease training loads to manage your total life stress, and then make sure that your recovery and nutrition are optimal. Of course, check with your doctor before embarking on this training plan. I strongly recommend you get some professional coaching to help you set up your workout plan and learn how to train in each zone safely and properly.

I've collected some examples of concurrent training plans used by elite athletes and coaches. One is from John Rogers, a swim coach from Australia who is currently heading up the High-Performance Swim Centre at the University of Toronto. He has consistently put his swimmers on the podium in several Olympic Games. His concurrent plan consists of a one-week cycle where the focus changes every 12 hours. He adapts this plan to emphasize different elements at different times of the year. For example, early in the season he places more emphasis on building endurance and higher total volumes, whereas later in the season he increases the amount of speed work leading up to competitions. But the week cycle rarely changes. John has been kind enough to let me reproduce his week plan here.

	MORNING	AFTERNOON/EVENING
MONDAY	Aerobic base + muscle-resistance training	Aerobic power
TUESDAY	Aerobic threshold + muscle-resistance training	Anaerobic training
WEDNESDAY	Aerobic threshold &/or power + muscle-resistance training	Off
THURSDAY	Workout changes depending on training plan + muscle-resistance training	Aerobic power
FRIDAY	Aerobic base and/or Power + muscle-resistance training	Anaerobic training
SATURDAY	Competition simulation	Off
SUNDAY	Off	Off

Below is another example of a concurrent training plan for a winter outdoor-sport training camp that a number of Olympians attended in January 2010. This plan was the one that Olympic gold medallist Adam van Koeverden used at a winter cross-training camp during his preparation for the 2011 competitive season. Although the template format is different, you can easily see how the training cycles through the various physiological demands.

	DAY	AM	PM	DATE	AM	PM
SUNDAY	1	Swimming 45 min EZ	Cross-country Skiing hour set	8	Swimming 45 min EZ	Cross-country Skiing hour set
MONDAY	2	Snowshoeing 3 hrs	Weights	9	Snowshoeing 3 hrs	Weights
TUESDAY	3	Running– Hard Intervals	Snowboarding / Skiing 4 hours	10	Spinning 60 min	Choice recovery activity 2 hours
WEDNESDAY	4	Weights	Cross-country Skiing hour set	11	Weights	Cross-country Skiing hour set
THURSDAY	5	Snowboarding / Skiing 4 hours	Weights	12	Snowboard / Skiing 4 hours	Weights
FRIDAY	6	OFF	Cross-country Skiing hour set	13	OFF	Cross-country Skiing hour set
SATURDAY	7	Weights	Snowboard / Ski 4 hours	14	Weights	Snowboarding / Skiing 4 hours

Green = Recovery exercise. Low to moderate heart rate. Maximum 90 minutes.
Yellow = Aerobic training. Moderate heart rate. Minimum 2 hours
Red = Aerobic-power training. Must do at least 40 minutes of maximum (10 or higher heart rate).

The final piece of the puzzle lies in how to best prepare for performance moments—how to perform on demand.

PERFORMANCE ON DEMAND: HOW WORLD-CLASS ATHLETES PERFORM WHEN IT MATTERS MOST

Imagine this scenario. You've been training for 10 years, each week working on your skills and physical abilities for at least 20 to 30 hours. That's several hours of focused, tough work every day for over a decade. And you've done all this for the chance to test yourself against other people who have trained just as hard as you. But you get only one chance. And this chance must happen on a specified day—in fact, at a specified time on that day. And you know that day and time years in advance. You know exactly when you'll have to perform, and you have to be at your peak. World-class athletes are specialists in such peak performances. They can't afford to "hope" that things will come together for them on a specific date at a specific time. They therefore have to employ specific techniques to supercharge their bodies and brains so that they get the most out of themselves right when they need to.

What would you be doing with 20 days to go until the start of an Olympic Games? Getting in lots of extra practice, hitting the gym to get just a bit stronger, maybe doing some additional cardio to make sure that

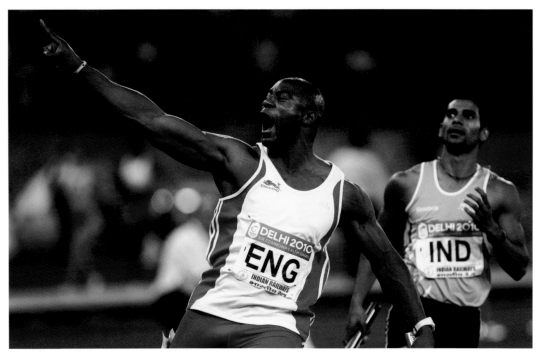

Before major competitions, athletes taper—decreasing their workload rather than increasing it. This sounds counterintuitive, but it actually produces a superior biological state that leads to optimal performance.

you are totally fit—right? Actually, most athletes do the exact opposite. World-class athletes follow a specific process just before competing. This process involves reducing the workload right before a performance. It's called tapering. More scientifically, tapering produces a superior biological state characterized by perfect health, a quick adaptability to training stimuli and a very high rate of recovery. Dr. Inigo Mujika from Spain (Twitter: @inigomujika_en) has defined taper as a "progressive non-linear reduction in the training load during a variable period of time, in an attempt to reduce the physiological and psychological stress of daily training and optimize sports performance."[85]

For about two or three weeks before major competitions, athletes typically *decrease* their amount of training and practice—sometimes by as much as 75%. During this period, they rest and relax as much as they can. So much so that a good friend of mine, Eddie Parenti—a captain of the Canadian Olympic swim team in the 1990s—would even refuse to walk up and down stairs before big meets. To quote him: "During taper season all bets are off for running, biking, weights, hoops—heck, even walking." And

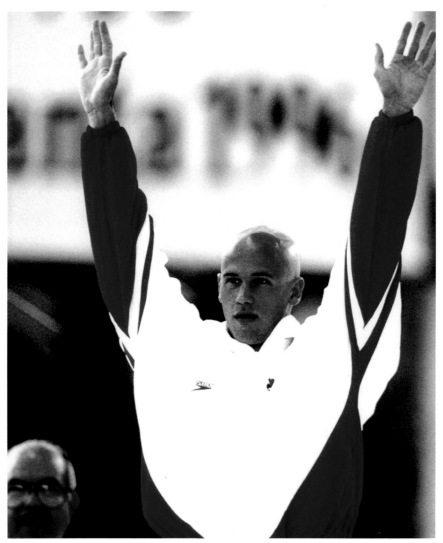

Eddie Parenti, Captain of Canada's Olympic swim team in the 1990s.

although it's completely opposite to what you'd expect athletes to be doing, it works brilliantly to improve performance by 2 to 4% in a matter of weeks. Such an improvement normally takes years to achieve if you keep training hard all the time. I have heard that tapering was discovered by accident in the early 1960s when a varsity swim team in the United States lost its pool because of an equipment malfunction for a week before a major competition. The swimmers could not practise, but when they went to the competition the entire team achieved their best times.

The primary objective of tapering is to decrease the training stress, thereby allowing the body to recover and eliminate fatigue. When the training impulse is decreased, fatigue decreases more rapidly than fitness; better performance results from the increasing difference between the two factors. Simply stated, when you are training hard, you are very fit—but you are also tired. As a result, your ability to perform at your best is limited by your fatigue. If you rest, however, your fatigue disappears very quickly, but your fitness decreases slowly. So when athletes taper, their goal is to get as much rest as quickly as possible to maximize the gap between fitness and fatigue. Then the challenge is to time the taper so that the maximum gap happens on the day of the competition. Start resting too soon, and your fitness decreases too much. But if you don't rest for long enough, you'll still feel the lingering effects of the preparatory training. In a well-designed taper, the body becomes rested (with all the associated benefits) and the athlete's fitness level is well maintained. When the training stress is decreased, the body assumes it has some time to make itself stronger, faster and fitter—so that when you start training again in the future, your body will be able to handle the stress more easily. All sorts of amazing things happen inside an athlete's body during taper—the blood improves, the muscles get stronger, the nervous system becomes more responsive and the psychological state gets better.

World-class athletes learn to use tapering to maximize their performance. But anyone can benefit from this practice. From runners who are training for races of any distance, to anyone getting ready for a big presentation at work, people can apply the taper principles to help their bodies perform at their best at the right time. Resting and decreasing the volume of practice or work before a concert, presentation or audition can improve your mental and physical capacities and help you perform at your best. In reality, resting for 3 weeks as world-class athletes do is not practical. But the effects can be felt in as little as 24 hours. So if you have a big event to prepare for, plan to have the 24 hours leading into it free so that you can rest and relax as needed.

I used this practice when I auditioned to be a commentator for the 2010 Olympics. A call had gone out for physiotherapists, doctors and scientists who were interested in being the on-camera host for a new series exploring the science of human performance during the Olympics. Of course, being a former competitive swimmer and now a scientist studying human physiology, I was excited about this opportunity to bring my knowledge of sport science to the Games.

The first audition was late in the day, so I went to work and then walked over to the studio afterward. I thought I had memorized the script, but after a long workday my focus had shifted to research rather than auditioning. I tried to perform well, but it was late in the day and I was tired after thinking intensely for 8 hours, so my performance on camera left a lot to be desired. I had trouble getting fired up, I was pretty nervous, I couldn't think clearly and I struggled. Thankfully, I was allowed several takes to get the read right, but I could tell the hiring committee was barely impressed. Nevertheless, I made it through the first cut. (I'm not exactly sure how, but I'll go with it.) I resolved to do much better the second time.

I decided to put all my experience as an athlete into helping me peak for the next on-camera performance. I memorized the script perfectly the weekend before the second audition, and then booked off work the day of the audition itself. This way, not only could I rest the night before instead of staying up late trying to learn lines when I was already sleepy, but I could also relax the day of the audition itself. The day of the call-back I did a light workout in the morning, followed by a low-carb, high-protein breakfast, which I know helps me to concentrate. I then took a bit of time to practise my lines before heading to the studio. I had a coffee 30 minutes before I was to speak on camera, and this time I nailed the performance. I could think clearly, I was happy and excited, and it felt great.

Tapering is a powerful tool that can help people from all walks of life to perform at a high level when they need to. It's a great example of how scientific discoveries from sport can be applied to other fields to improve health and performance. Try it the next time you have to take part in a running race, give a big presentation or write an exam.

THE LAST WORD

I spend most of my working life with incredible people. When I was swimming competitively I trained with many athletes who were representing their countries in the Olympics. I was taught by some fantastic coaches, all of whom had a great influence on me. I learned from the very best professors, doctors and scientists in my academic life. As an instructor at the National Coaching Institute, I've provided feedback and suggestions for many of the best coaches in their respective sports. The swimmers that I've coached and the athletes that I've worked with have helped me understand how important knowledge is and just how far passion and focus can take us. But the most powerful lessons I've learned have come from children. I've been able to do research with some wonderful patients and their families at the Toronto Hospital for Sick Children and I have seen children deal with cancer with happiness and hope.

Committing to a well-designed exercise program supported by innovative ideas is one of the most important things you can do to experience a healthy and happy life. In this book I've described how your heart, lungs and blood work together to provide the energy you need to stay healthy and perform well. I've talked about how muscles work, and how important strength training is. I've found that when the athletes I worked with understood why they were exercising in a certain way their effort and motivation for training improved tremendously. I hope that this is the case for you as well.

To support your new exercise and training activities, consider the information I've presented about the immune and endocrine systems. Think of what I've said about how to recover after exercise or other life stresses. The

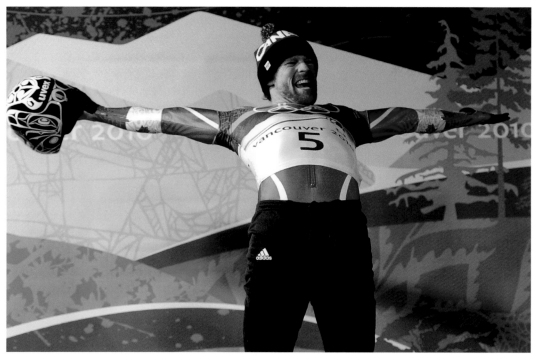

Jon Montgomery celebrating his gold medal win at the Vancouver Olympics.

practices in this book can help you stay healthy and manage your mental and physical state on a daily basis.

Nutrition is the foundation of human health and performance, and I've placed key information about nutrition throughout the book to help you eat well as you face any challenges in the future.

I've covered all the main organ systems in the human body, and your new understanding of how these systems work when the body is pushed to its limits will help you achieve higher performance in sports and a life that is full of health and happiness. To achieve this high level of performance and health you need to take advantage of the power of goal setting and its influence on human motivation.

I was speaking about this very subject at a TEDx conference in Toronto in the months following the 2010 Olympics. (If you are not familiar with the TED talks, check them out at www.ted.com.) The audience was made up mostly of children from schools from all over North America. In my talk I spoke about what had made Olympians successful at the recent Games. I showed how Petra Majdic won a bronze medal in cross-country skiing, after breaking ribs and suffering a pneumothorax in warm-up, by relying on her passion for her sport. I talked about Joannie Rochette and her incredible ability to stay focused on her skating routine despite having tragically lost her mother only days before the Olympics. Then I moved on to Jon Montgomery, the skeleton racer who won a gold medal and then proceeded to enjoy one of the more memorable celebrations I've ever seen. His furious fist-pumping, his jump on to the podium and his celebratory walk through Whistler are now legendary.

At this point in my talk I showed a picture of Jon taken right after he realized he had won the medal. All 500 children in the audience were smiling and following my words closely as I talked about the look on Jon's face. His exhilaration, relief and pride were evident in every pixel of the photograph. I showed the audience pictures of other great champions: Usain Bolt, Adam Van Koeverden, Mark Tewksbury. They all had the same look on their faces. I explained to the audience that these dedicated athletes have committed themselves completely to reaching their goals. The joy on their faces is evidence of how it feels to achieve the things that you strive for in life. At this point, the audience was quiet, so I paused as well. I turned around and looked at the picture of Jon Montgomery on the podium, and spoke a thought out loud: "I don't get to feel like that at work very often." Everyone laughed. "Maybe goals aren't enough," I added. The audience was paying close attention. Thinking out loud again, I said, "Maybe this concept of goal-setting is not the most powerful of all. . . . These people haven't just achieved their goals; they've achieved their DREAMS." The audience cheered at these words.

This was the powerful thought that captured everyone's imagination that day. The kids in the audience had led me to the most important idea in my entire speech. It was the only part of the speech that people tweeted about.

We need to develop a new concept. Forget goal-setting—we need *dream-setting*. Martin Luther King, who dreamed about civil rights; Ghandi, who dreamed about truth; and Mother Theresa, who dreamed about love—they all changed the world.

I have a dream as well. I dream that we will all understand and appreciate the wonder of the human body. I dream of a time when we can use exercise as therapy to cure disease. I dream of athletes using physiological science to push the limits of human achievement. And I dream that you can use the information in this book to improve your life, even if it is by as little as 1%.

—Greg Wells, Ph.D.

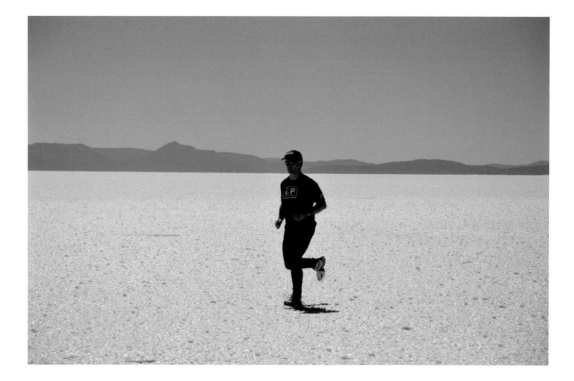

ACKNOWLEDGEMENTS

I am so lucky to have had awe-inspiring people in my life who have provided me with many rich opportunities to learn and enabled me to experience so much of what this world has to offer. Throughout this book I've included photos, stories and information from friends, family and many respected colleagues. This book is intensely personal and I could never have done anything in my life—much less write these pages—without the support and human interactions that have created the experiences referenced herein.

My academic career has had many ups and downs, but there are some key people who have helped me at critical points, specifically Pat Mills, Doug Smith, Dr. Monika Schloder, Dr. Michael Plyley, Dr. James Duffin, Dr. Allan Coates, Dr. Ingrid Tein and Dr. Joe Fisher. Thank you for your support and patience, and in some cases a hard kick in the butt.

During the writing of this volume, I relied heavily on my colleagues Doug Vanderby and Donna Wilkes and my science mentor, Dr. James Duffin. Your insights and comments were invaluable. I also want to thank my literary agent, Chris Bucci, from Anne McDermid and Associates, for contacting me after the 2010 Olympics and making this dream a reality. My editor, Brad Wilson, from HarperCollins Publishers, played a significant role in helping to direct the focus of this book. And for taking me on as an author, I thank you!

The content of *Superbodies* is based on my experiences working and playing at the physical extremes, both in good times and bad. I've had the privilege of working with amazing athletes, inspirational coaches and wonderful children and families at the Hospital for Sick Children. I've trained with the most fun and positive people you could ever hope to have as teammates. None of what I have learned and experienced would have been possible without you. Thanks for being such an important part of my life. I hope that I have presented your stories respectfully and accurately.

I'd like to thank CTV, TSN, Sportsnet and ABC for having me as their sports science analyst during the Olympic Broadcasts, and Peace Point Entertainment Group for having me as the host and science consultant for the *Superbodies* segments that aired during the Olympics. The computer-generated images that appear in these pages were drawn from those segments and I am honoured that they are part of this work.

Every once in a while I find the time to sit back and think about my life and my experiences. Each time I do this the most important people who come to mind are my original family—my mom and dad; and Sarah, Brent and Declan—and my new family, Theresa, Chris and Margaret. I am so lucky to be a part of both these families. I love you all very much.

Finally, to my wonderful wife, Judith, and my baby girl, Ingrid, who I love more than life itself (and I love life a lot!). You are my world. This book, along with everything else I do, is for you.

NOTES

INTRODUCTION: WORKING SMARTER, NOT HARDER

*   C.P. Wen, J.P. Wai, M.K. Tsai, Y.C. Yang, T.Y. Cheng, M.C. Lee, H.T. Chan, C.K. Tsao, S.P. Tsai, X. Wu, "Minimize Amount of Physical Activity for Reduced Mortality and Extended Life Expectancy: A Prospective Cohort Study," *The Lancet* (August 16, 2011).

CHAPTER 1: FUELLING YOUR BODY

1   P. Radermacher, K. J. Falke, Y. S. Park, D. W. Ahn, S. K. Hong, J. Qvist, and W. M. Zapol, "Nitrogen Tensions in Brachial Vein Blood of Korean Ama Divers," *Journal of Applied Physiology* 73 (1992): 2592–5.

2   Jerome A. Dempsey, A. William Sheel, Claudette M. St Croix, and Barbara J. Morgan, "Respiratory Influences on Sympathetic Vasomotor Outflow in Humans," *Respiratory Physiology & Neurobiology* 130, no. 1 (March 2002): 3–20.

3   I. Mujika, S. Padilla, A. Geyssant, and J. C. Chatard, "Hematological Responses to Training and Taper in Competitive Swimmers: Relationships with Performance," *Archives of Physiology and Biochemistry* 105, no. 4 (August 1998): 379–85.

4   G. Q. Zhang and W. Zhang, "Heart Rate, Lifespan, and Mortality Risk," *Ageing Research Reviews* 8, no. 1 (January 2009): 52–60. Epub edition.

5   Peter Woodford, "Are Sports Bad for the Ticker?" *National Review of Medicine* 3, no. 1 (January 2006).

6   J. A. Drezner and K. J. Rogers, "Sudden Cardiac Arrest in Intercollegiate Athletes: Detailed Analysis and Outcomes of Resuscitation in Nine Cases," *Heart Rhythm* 3, no. 7 (July 2006): 755–9. Epub edition.

CHAPTER 2: POWERING HUMAN MOVEMENT

7   G. D. Wells, H. Selvadurai, and I. Tein, "Bioenergetic Provision of Energy for Muscular Activity," *Paediatric Respiratory Reviews* 10, no. 3 (September 2009): 83–90. Epub edition.

8   A. Bonen, "Lactate Transporters (MCT Proteins) in Heart and Skeletal Muscles," *Medicine & Science in Sports & Exercise* 32, no. 4 (April 2000): 778–89.

9   S. Trappe, D. Costill, and R. Thomas, "Effect of Swim Taper on Whole Muscle and Single Fiber Contractile Properties," *Medicine & Science in Sports & Exercise* 32 (2000): 48–56.

10   D. E. Lieberman, M. Venkadesan, W. A. Werbel, A. I. Daoud, S. D'Andrea, I. S. Davis, R. O. Mang'eni, and Y. Pitsiladis, "Foot Strike Patterns and Collision Forces in Habitually Barefoot versus Shod Runners," *Nature* 463, no. 7280 (January 28, 2010): 531–5.

11   G. D. Wells, D. L. Wilkes, J. E. Schneiderman, T. Rayner, M. Elmi, H. Selvadurai, S. Dell, M. D. Noseworthy, F. Ratjen, I. Tein, and A. L. Coates, "Skeletal Muscle Metabolism in Cystic Fibrosis and Primary Ciliary Dyskinesia," *Pediatric Research* 69, no. 1 (January 2011): 40–45.

12   P. J. Vignos Jr. and M. P. Watkins, "The Effect of Exercise in Muscular Dystrophy," *Journal of the American Medical Association* 197, no. 11 (September 12, 1966): 843–8.

13   Marie Louise Sveen, Tina D. Jeppesen, Simon Hauerslev, Lars Køber, Thomas O. Krag, and John Vissing, "Endurance Training Improves Fitness and Strength in Patients with Becker Muscular Dystrophy," *Brain: A Journal of Neurology* 131, no. 11 (2008), 2824–31.

14   F. H. Nielsen and H.C. Lukaski, "Update on the Relationship between Magnesium and Exercise," *Magnesium Research* 19, no. 3 (September 2006):180–9.

15   E. Jean-St-Michel, C. Manlhiot, J. Li, M. Tropak, M. M. Michelsen, M. R. Schmidt, B. W. McCrindle, G. D. Wells, and A.N. Redington, "Remote Preconditioning Improves Maximal Performance in Highly Trained Athletes," *Medicine & Science in Sports & Exercise* 43, no. 7 (July 2011): 1280–6.

16   G. Wahi, P.C. Parkin, J. Beyene, E.M. Uleryk, C.S. Birkin, "Effectiveness of Interventions Aimed at Reducing Screen Time in Children: A Systematic Review and Meta-analysis of Randomized Controlled Trials," *Archives of Pediatrics and Adolescent Medicine* 165, no. 11 (November 2011): 979–86.

CHAPTER 3: ENERGIZING YOUR BRAIN

17   K. Zukor and Z. He, "Regenerative Medicine: Drawing Breath after Spinal Injury," *Nature* 475 no. 7355 (July 13, 2011):177–8.

18   Check out Norman Doidge's book at www.normandoidge.com.

19   A. C. Pereira, D. E. Huddleston, A. M. Brickman, A. A. Sosunov, R. Hen, G. M. McKhann, R. Sloan, F. H. Gage, T. R. Brown, and S. A. Small, "An In Vivo Correlate of Exercise-Induced Neurogenesis in the Adult Dentate Gyrus," *Proceedings of the National Academy of Sciences of the United States of America* 104, no. 13 (March 27, 2007): 5638–43. Epub edition.

20   E. B. Larson, L. Wang, J. D. Bowen, W. C. McCormick, L. Teri, P. Crane, and W. Kukull, "Exercise Is Associated with Reduced Risk for Incident Dementia among Persons 65 Years of Age and Older," *Annals of Internal Medicine* 144, no. 2 (January 17, 2006):73–81.

21   C. H. Hillman, M. B. Pontifex, L. B. Raine, D. M. Castelli, E. E. Hall, A. F. Kramer. "The Effect of Acute Treadmill Walking on Cognitive Control and Academic Achievement in Preadolescent Children," *Neuroscience* 159, no. 3 (March 31, 2009):1044–54.

22   A. Gill, R. Womack, and S. Safranek, "Clinical Inquiries: Does Exercise Alleviate Symptoms of Depression?" *Journal of Family Practice* 59, no. 9 (September 2010): 530–1.

23 J. A. Blumenthal, "New Frontiers in Cardiovascular Behavioral Medicine: Comparative Effectiveness of Exercise and Medication in Treating Depression," *Cleveland Clinic Journal of Medicine* 78, no. S1 (August 2011): S35–S43.

24 Douglass L, "Yoga as an Intervention in the Treatment of Eating Disorders: Does It Help?" *Eating Disorders* 17 (2009): 126–139.

25 A. Ross and S. Thomas, "The Health Benefits of Yoga and Exercise: A Review of Comparison Studies," Journal of Alternative and Complementary Medicine 16, no. 1 (January 2010): 3–12.

26 Britta K. Hölzel, James Carmody, Mark Vangel, Christina Congleton, Sita M. Yerramsetti, Tim Gard, and Sara W. Lazar, "Mindfulness Practice Leads to Increases in Regional Brain Grey Matter Density," *Psychiatry Research: Neuroimaging* 191, no. 1 (January 2011): 36–43.

27 R. J. Maddock, A. S. Garrett, and M. H. Buonocore, "Posterior Cingulate Cortex Activation by Emotional Words: MRI Evidence from a Valence Decision Task," *Human Brain Mapping* 18, no 1 (January 2003): 30–41.

28 R. Saxe and N. Kanwisher, "People Thinking about Thinking People: The Role of the Temporo-Parietal Junction in 'theory of mind,' *Neuroimage* 19, no. 4 (August 2003): 1835–42.

29 T. Low Dog, "The Role of Nutrition in Mental Health," *Alternative Therapies in Health and Medicine* 16, no. 2 (March 2010): 42–6.

30 T. N. Akbaraly, E. J. Brunner, J. E. Ferrie, M. G. Marmot, M. Kivimaki, and A. Singh-Manoux, "Dietary Pattern and Depressive Symptoms in Middle Age," *British Journal of Psychiatry* 195, no. 5 (November 2009): 408–13.

31 A. Sánchez-Villegas, M. Delgado-Rodríguez, A. Alonso, J. Schlatter, F. Lahortiga, L. Serra Majem, and M. A. Martínez-González, "Association of the Mediterranean Dietary Pattern with the Incidence of Depression: the Seguimiento Universidad de Navarra/University of Navarra Follow-up (SUN) Cohort," *Archives of General Psychiatry* 66, no. 10 (October 2009): 1090–8.

32 C. A. Salter, "Dietary Tyrosine as an Aid to Stress Resistance among Troops," *Military Medicine* 154, no. 3 (March 1989): 144–6.

33 E. S. Chambers, M. W. Bridge, and D. A. Jones, "Carbohydrate Sensing in the Human Mouth: Effects on Exercise Performance and Brain Activity," *Journal of Physiology* 587, Pt 8 (April 2009): 1779–94.

CHAPTER 4: RESISTING ILLNESS AND DISEASE

34 E. A. Murphy, J. M. Davis, M. D. Carmichael, J. D. Gangemi, A. Ghaffar, and E. P. Mayer, "Exercise Stress Increases Susceptibility to Influenza Infection," *Brain, Behavior, and Immunity* 22, no. 8 (November 2008): 1152–5. Epub edition.

35 H. B. Simon, "The Immunology of Exercise: A Brief Review," *Journal of the American Medical Association* 252, no. 19 (November 1984): 2735–8.

36 David C. Nieman, "Marathon Training and Immune Function," Sports Medicine 37 (2007): 412–415.

37 M. Gleeson and D. B. Pyne, "Special Feature for the Olympics: Effects of Exercise on the Immune System: Exercise Effects on Mucosal Immunity," *Immunology & Cell Biology* 75, no. 5 (October 2000): 536–44.

38   A. Moreira, F. Arsati, P. R. Cury, C. Franciscon, P. R. de Oliveira, and V. C. de Araújo, "Salivary Immunoglobulin a Response to a Match in Top-Level Brazilian Soccer Players," *Journal of Strength & Conditioning Research* 23, no. 7 (October 2009): 1968–73.

39   N. P. Walsh, M. Gleeson, D. B. Pyne, D. C. Nieman, F. S. Dhabhar, R. J. Shephard, S. J. Oliver, S. Bermon, and A. Kajeniene, "Position Statement. Part Two: Maintaining Immune Health," *Exercise Immunology Review* 17 (2011): 64–103.

40   E. M. Peters, "Exercise, Immunology and Upper Respiratory Tract Infections," *International Journal of Sports Medicine* 18, no. S1 (March 1997): S69–77.

41   K. I. Block and M. N. Mead, "Immune System Efects of Echinacea, Ginseng and Astragalus: A Review," *Integrative Cancer Therapies* 2, no. 3 (September 2003): 247–67.

42   K. Linde K, B. Barrett, K. Wölkart, R. Bauer, D. Melchart, "Echinacea for Preventing and Treating the Common Cold," *Cochrane Database Systematic Reviews* 25, no. 1 (January 2006):CD000530.

43   I. Mujika, J. C. Chatard, and A. Geyssant, "Effects of Training and Taper on Blood Leucocyte Populations in Competitive Swimmers: Relationships with Cortisol and Performance," *International Journal of Sports Medicine* 17 (1996): 213–7.

44   R. M. Douglas and H. Hemilä, "Vitamin C for Preventing and Treating the Common Cold," *PLoS Medicine* 2, no. 6 (June 2005): e168; quiz e217. Epub edition.

45   A. K. Blannin, P. J. Robson, N. P. Walsh, A. M. Clark, L. Glennon, M. Gleeson, "The Effect of Exercising to Exhaustion at Different Intensities on Saliva Immunoglobulin A, Protein and Electrolyte Secretion," *International Journal of Sports Medicine* 19, no. 8 (November 1998): 547–52.

46   R. Chandra, "Nutrition and the Immune System: An Introduction," *American Journal of Clinical Nutrition* 66 (1997): 460S-3S.

47   N. Chainani-Wu, "Safety and Anti-Inflammatory Activity of Curcumin: A Component of Turmeric (Curcuma longa)," *Journal of Alternative and Complementary Medicine* 9, no. 1 (February 2003): 161–8.

48   S. C. Segerstrom and G. E. Miller, "Psychological Stress and the Human Immune System: A Meta-Analytic Study of 30 Years of Inquiry," *Psychological Bulletin* 130, no. 4 (July 2004): 601–30.

49   M. Gleeson, J. L. Francis, D. J. Lugg, R. L. Clancy, J. M. Ayton, J.A. Reynolds, and C. A. McConnell, "One Year in Antarctica: Mucosal Immunity at Three Australian Stations," *Immunology & Cell Biology* 78, no. 6 (December 2000): 616–22.

50   Segerstrom et al.

51   E. M. Reiche, S. O. Nunes, H. K. Morimoto, "Stress, Depression, the Immune System, and Cancer," Lancet Oncology 5, no. 10 (October 2004): 617–25.

52   C. J. Rogers, L. H. Colbert, J. W. Greiner, S. N. Perkins, and S. D. Hursting, "Physical Activity and Cancer Prevention: Pathways and Targets for Intervention," Sports Medicine 38, no. 4 (2008): 271–96.

53   http://www.nature.com/bjc/journal/v100/n4/abs/6604917a.html

CHAPTER 5: PERFORMING UNDER PRESSURE

54   I. Mujika, S. Padilla, D. Pyne, and T. Busso, "Physiological Changes Associated with the Pre-Event Taper in Athletes," *Sports Medicine* 34, no. 13 (2004): 891–927.

55   Henriksen, E. J., "Exercise Training and the Antioxidant Alpha-Lipoic Acid in the Treatment of Insulin Resistance and Type 2 Diabetes," *Free Radical Biology & Medicine* 40, no. 1 (January 1, 2006): 3–12.

56   J. P. Henry, "Biological Basis of the Stress Response," *News in Psychological Sciences* 8 (1993): 69–73.

57   E. Epel, R. Lapidus, B. McEwen, et al, "Stress May Add Bite to Appetite in Women: A Laboratory Study of Stress-Induced Cortisol and Eating Behaviour," *Psychoneuroendocrinology* 26 (2001): 37–49.

58   Henning Boecker, Till Sprenger, Mary E. Spilker, Gjermund Henriksen, Marcus Koppenhoefer, Klaus J. Wagner, Michael Valet, Achim Berthele, and Thomas R. Tolle, "The Runner's High: Opioidergic Mechanisms in the Human Brain," *Cerebral Cortex* 18, no. 11 (November 2008): 2523–2531, doi:10.1093/cercor/bhn013.

59   S. R. Taylor, G. G. Rogers, and H. S. Driver, "Effects of Training Volume on Sleep, Psychological, and Selected Physiological Profiles of Elite Female Swimmers," *Medicine & Science in Sports & Exercise* 29 (1997): 688–93.

60   P. J. Jenkins, A. Mukherjee, and S. M. Shalet, "Does Growth Hormone Cause Cancer?" *Clinical Endocrinology* (Oxford) 64, no. 2 (February 2006): 115–21.

61   T. Oosthuyse and A. N. Bosch, "The Effect of the Menstrual Cycle on Exercise Metabolism: Implications for Exercise Performance in Eumenorrhoeic Women," *Sports Medicine* 40, no. 3 (March 2010): 207–27.

62   X. A. Janse de Jonge, "Effects of the Menstrual Cycle on Exercise Performance," *Sports Medicine* 33, no. 11 (2003): 833–51.

63   B. L. Drinkwater, B. Bruemner, and C. H. Chesnut III, "Menstrual History as a Determinant of Current Bone Density in Young Athletes," *Journal of the American Medical Association* 263, no. 4 (January 1990): 545–8.

CHAPTER 6: PERFORMANCE CYCLING

64   U. Hartmann and J. Mester, "Training and Overtraining Markers in Selected Sport Events," *Medicine & Science in Sports & Exercise* 32, no. 1 (January 2000): 209–15.

65   W. C. McMaster, T. Stoddard, and W. Duncan, "Enhancement of Blood Lactate Clearance Following Maximal Swimming. Effect of Velocity of Recovery Swimming," *American Journal of Sports Medicine* 17, no. 4 (July-August 1989): 472–7.

66   J. Vescovi, O. Falenchuk, and G. D. Wells, "Blood Lactate Concentration and Clearance in Elite Swimmers During Competition," *International Journal of Sports Physiology and Performance* 6, no. 1 (March 2011): 106–17.

67   J. L. Ivy, A. L. Katz, C. L. Cutler, W. M. Sherman, and E. F. Coyle, "Muscle Glycogen Synthesis After Exercise: Effect of Time of Carbohydrate Ingestion," *Journal of Applied Physiology* 64 (1988): 1480–1485.

68   Paul J. Flakoll, Tom Judy, Kim Flinn, Christopher Carr, and Scott Flinn, "Postexercise Protein Supplementation Improves Health and Muscle Soreness During Basic Military Training in Marine Recruits," *Journal of Applied Physiology* 96 (2004): 951–956.

69   Gatorade Sport Science Institute Sport Science Exchange Roundtable # 46, "Speeding Recovery from Exercise," Volume 12, no. 4 (2001). http://www.gssiweb.com/ Article_Detail.aspx?articleid=297&level=2&topic=17

70   Deanna K. Levenhagen, Jennifer D. Gresham, Michael G. Carlson, David J. Maron, Myfanwy J. Borel, and Paul J. Flakoll, "Post-Exercise Nutrient Intake Timing in Humans is Critical to Recovery of Leg Glucose, Homeostasis," *American Journal of Physiology: Endocrinology and Metabolism* 280, no. 6 (2001): E982–993.

71   C. M. Bleakley and G. W. Davison, "What is the Biochemical and Physiological Rationale for Using Cold-Water Immersion in Sports Recovery? A Systemic Review," *British Journal of Sports Medicine* 44, no. 3 (February 2010): 179–87.

72   J. R. Jakeman, R. Macrae, and R. Eston, "A Single 10-minute Bout of Cold-Water Immersion Therapy After Strenuous Plyometric Exercise Has No Beneficial Effect on Recovery from the Symptoms of Exercise-Induced Muscle Damage," *Ergonomics* 52, no. 4 (April 2009): 456–60.

73   H. Al Haddad, P. B. Laursen, D. Chollet, F. Lemaitre, S. Ahmaidi, and M. Buchheit, "Effect of Cold or Thermoneutral Water Immersion on Post-Exercise Heart Rate Recovery and Heart Rate Variability Indices," *Autonomic Neuroscience* 156, no 1–2 (August 25, 2010): 111–6.

74   H. Pournot, F. Bieuzen, R. Duffield, P. M. Lepretre, C. Cozzolino, and C. Hausswirth, "Short- Term Effects of Various Water Immersions on Recovery from Exhaustive Intermittent Exercise," *European Journal of Applied Physiology.* Epub edition.

75   J. R. Jakeman, C. Byrne, and R. G. Eston, "Lower-Limb Compression Garment Improves Recovery from Exercise-Induced Muscle Damage in Young, Active Females," European Journal of Applied Physiology 109, no. 6 (August 2010): 1137–44.

76   A. T. Scanlan, B. J. Dascombe, P. R. Reaburn, and M. Osborne, "The Effects of Wearing Lower-Body Compression Garments During Endurance Cycling," *International Journal of Sports Physiology and Performance* 3, no. 4 (December 2008): 424–38.

77   A. Ali, R. H. Creasy, and J. A. Edge, "Physiological Effects of Wearing Graduated Compression Stockings During Running," *European Journal of Applied Physiology.* Epub edition.

78   B. Sperlich, M. Haegele, S. Achtzehn, J. Linville, H. C. Holmberg, and J. Mester, "Different Types of Compression Clothing Do Not Increase Sub-Maximal and Maximal Endurance Performance in Well-Trained Athletes," *Journal of Sports Sciences* 28, no. 6 (April 2010): 609–14.

79   E. V. Wiltshire, V. Poitras, M. Pak, T. Hong, J. Rayner, and M. E. Tschakovsky, "Massage Impairs Postexercise Muscle Blood Flow and "Lactic Acid" Removal," *Medicine & Science in Sports & Exercise* 42, no. 6 (June 2010): 1062–71.

80   P. Weerapong, P. A. Hume, and G. S. Kolt, "The Mechanisms of Massage and Effects on Performance, Muscle Recovery and Injury Prevention," *Sports Medicine* 35, no. 3 (2005): 235–56.

81   J. D. Crane, D. I. Ogborn, C. Cupido, S. Melov, A. Hubbard, J. M. Bourgeois, and M. A. Tarnopolsky, "Massage Therapy Attenuates Inflammatory Signaling After Exercise-Induced Muscle Damage," *Science Translation Medicine* 4, no. 119 (February 2012): 119–13.

82   K. Baar, "Training for Endurance and Strength: Lessons from Cell Signalling," *Medicine & Science in Sports & Exercise* 38, no. 11 (November 2006): 1939–44.

83   G. A. Nader, "Concurrent Strength and Endurance Training: From Molecules to Man," *Medicine & Science in Sports & Exercise* 38, no. 11 (November 2006): 1965–70.

84   M. L. Walsh, "Whole-Body Fatigue and Critical Power: A Physiological Interpretation," *Sports Medicine* 29, no. 3 (March 2000): 153–66.

85   I. Mujika and S. Padilla, "Scientific Bases for Pre-Competition Tapering Strategies," *Medicine & Science in Sports & Exercise* 35, no. 7 (July 2003): 1182–7.

SOURCES

Borek, C. "Dietary Antioxidants and Human Cancer." *Integrated Cancer Therapies* 3, no. 4 (2004): 333–41.

Burke, L. "Nutrition for Recovery after Training and Competition." In *Clinical Sports Nutrition,* 3rd edition, edited by L. Burke and V. Deakin. Australia: McGraw-Hill, 2006.

Clarke, R., Armitage, J. "Antioxidant Vitamins and Risk of Cardiovascular Disease: Review of Large-Scale Randomised Trials." *Cardiovascular Drugs and Therapy* 16, no. 5 (September 2002): 411–5.

Feng, W. Y. "Metabolism of Green Tea Catechins: An Overview." *Current Drug Metabolism* 7, no. 7 (October 2006): 755–809.

Horrigan, L. A., J. P. Kelly, and T. J. Connor. "Immunomodulatory Effects of Caffeine: Friend or Foe?" *Pharmacology & Therapeutics* 111, no. 3 (September 2006): 877–92. Epub edition.

Huang, H. Y., B. Caballero, S. Chang, A. Alberg, R. Semba, C. Schneyer, R. F. Wilson, T. Y. Cheng, G. Prokopowicz, G. J. Barnes 2nd, J. Vassy, and E. B. Bass. "Multivitamin/Mineral Supplements and Prevention of Chronic Disease." *Evidence Report/Technology Assessment* no. 139 (May 2006): 1–117.

Reynolds, E. "Vitamin B12, Folic Acid, and the Nervous System." *The Lancet Neurology* 5, no. 11 (November 2006): 949–60.

Rahman, I. "Antioxidant Therapies in COPD." *International Journal of Chronic Obstructive Pulmonary Disease* 1, no. 1 (2006): 15–29.

Ratey, John. *Spark: The Revolutionary New Science of Exercise and the Brain.* New York: Little, Brown, 2008.

Osho. *Meditation: The First and Last Freedom.* New York: St. Martin's Griffin, 1997.

INDEX

erythroprotein (EPO), 13, 16–17

estrogen, 154

eustress (good stress), 139–42

exercise. *See also* specific topics
 best time of day for, 192
 improves health at any age, 85
 intensity, 9

fast-twitch fibres, 33–34

fat, 55

fatigue, 162
 extreme, 41–46
 fighting, 79–81

"female athlete triad," 155

fight-or-flight response, 136–37

Fisher, Joe, 14

force, defined, 53

free diving, 5–9

GABA (gamma-aminobutyric acid), 72

Gage, Fred, 84

Gleeson, Marie, 122–23

GLUT-4 (glucose transporter type 4), 157

glutathione, 26. *See also* N-acetyl-L-cysteine

glycogen, 38, 173–76

glycolysis, 38

glycolytic system and fibres, 32–36, 38, 202

golgi tendon organ (GTO), 77, 78

Goode, Robert, 9

green tea, 118

Griffin, Andrew, 45

growth hormone. *See* human growth hormone

gymnasts, 79

H1N1 (Influenza A virus subtype H1N1), 106, 107

Hamilton, Robert, 24

He, Zhigang, 70

heart. *See also* cardiovascular system
 oxygen and the, 19–24

heart attack, sudden death from, 23–24

heart rate (HR), 88–89, 94, 107, 171, 172, 200, 201, 214. *See also* heart; Rusko test
 how to use it to control training, 20
 measuring, 183–84
 resting, 20–21, 183–85

heart-rate variability (HRV), 88–89

heart safety during exercise, 23

heat, how the body adapts to, 2, 44–46

Hemilä, Harry, 111

herbal remedies, 108

high-energy phosphate (HEP) capacity and power-zone training, 204–5

hippocampus, 84

Holden, Jody, 89–90

hormones. See also endocrine system
 changes with rest, 134–36

Hospital for Sick Children in Toronto, 5, 24, 47, 55, 117, 133, 219, 223

hot temperatures. *See* heat

Humanetics training model, 189. *See also* specific topics

human growth hormone (HGH), 152–53

hydration, 168–70

hypothalamic-pituitary-adrenal (HPA) axis, 132, 136, 137

hypothalamus, 133

hypothermia, 46. *See also* cold temperatures

hypoxic ventilatory response (HVR), 14–16

INDEX